Every

OPTIMIZED PATIENT

Knows...

- Why a medical success is different than a clinical success, and why you need both to achieve a successful surgery and live a pain-free life.
- How surgeons watch closely for a patient's "will to get well" because they know it is key to thriving after spine surgery.
- How the appropriate use of painkillers can help you get critically needed restorative rest essential to sustainable healing.
- Why fear is the trap that keeps millions of people living in endless chronic pain.
- How to eat your way to a full recovery with fresh food programmed to restart your microbiome, giving your body the phyto-chemicals it needs to heal rapidly.
- Why therapeutic exercise and physical therapy are essential to your full recovery because healing oxygen and nutrients are delivered by active blood flow.
- Why and how aqua-therapy can be your secret weapon to avoid spine surgery altogether.

THE

OPTIMIZED PATIENT

2.0

Harvey Warren

Revised and expanded

OPTIMIZED OUTCOME SOLUTIONS

DIGITAL LEGEND

ISBN-13: 978-1-937735-24-1
Published by Digital Legend Press & Publishing, Inc.
Salt Lake City, Utah

Inquiries or Permissions: info@digitalegend.com or by phone: 801-810-7718
Cover and interior design by Jacob F. Frandsen
Printed in the United States of America

With love and gratitude to my precious wife, who is the world's most patient caregiver and my relentless cheerleader.

May all who read this book be blessed by such a one as she.

CONTENTS

Foreword ix
Author's Note xix
1. It's A Commitment. 1
2. You Are Not Alone 17
3. What Happened? 35
4. What Are My Options?. 53
5. Fear and Denial. 69
6. The Surgeons' Perspective. .87
7. Why Optimize? 105
8. Know What To Ask . . . Before 123
9. Win Or Lose In Rehab 141
10. The Will To Get Well 161
11. Fire Up The Recovery Engine! 179
12. Becoming You Again 199
Addendum for Caregivers 217
Afterword 229

FOREWORD

by Bill Walton

Can you count on one hand how many people who have changed the direction of your life? During the writing of this book I was fortunate to add another friend to my list, Bill Walton.

Bill is a retired American basketball player and current television sportscaster. He achieved superstardom playing for John Wooden's powerhouse UCLA Bruins in the early '70s and winning three straight College Player of the Year Awards, and he went on to have a prominent career in the NBA. Walton was inducted into the Basketball Hall of Fame on May 10, 1993 and the Oregon Sports Hall of Fame that same year.

As you will read in this powerful and heartfelt foreword, Bill Walton was able to overcome crippling back pain and change the direction of his life. The wisdom he shared with me changed the direction of mine. His message, our message is simple, "if we can do it, you can do it too." With Bill's permission I now share his thoughts with you and ask that you pay it forward to anyone willing to scale the terrible mountain that is chronic back pain.

CLIMBING TO THE TOP OF THE MOUNTAIN—ONE MORE TIME

Talk is cheap.

Particularly when it comes to throwing around the sports clichés that capture our desperate infatuation with recovery.

The turnaround. The rebound. Starting the fast-break. Transition. The climb beats the descent.

It all seems so easy. Say a few words, and all of a sudden you're back on track in the game of life.

The long hard climb is really the easy part. Getting on or into it is what is so frighteningly elusive and difficult.

I know. I've been there. And until you've been there yourself—you really have no idea.

I know. I had no idea.

I've been on top before. And it's definitely the place to be.

Success came early and easy to me in my world of basketball and academics. I had a better than perfect childhood of fairy tale quality.

Growing up in a completely non-athletic family, I was fortunate to have parents who loved me more than they cared about themselves. I had teachers and coaches who thoroughly enjoyed their critical roles in helping develop other people's lives and dreams. And I had heroes across the board who genuinely lived and played in the game of life with passion and purpose. They lived like they talked, and they dreamed they were going to the top.

The influential adults in my life as a young boy growing up in San Diego stood for more than material accumulation of stuff; for more than physical gratification.

Adversity is a constant in life, although I certainly was not aware of any serious hardship as a child. I did though, grow up thinking that everybody's feet hurt all the time and that only the lucky ones could talk. Later on I came to believe that everybody's back hurt all the time too—and that foot and back pain were all just a part of the way things are.

I was born with structural, congenital defects in my feet. I am a life-long stutterer. I broke my spine playing basketball for UCLA when I was 21 years old.

These factors have all played significant roles throughout my life with the many daunting twists that fate delivers to your door.

I was on a big roll and run at UCLA in the early 1970's before being low-bridged in a despicable act of violence and dirty play that caused me to fracture some bones in my back. 12 days later I lost the next game that I played in—the first loss in nearly 5 years. I lost a lot more than just a basketball game that day. It takes a lot to win, even more to lose.

A few years later I was the reigning NBA Champion and league MVP. Those structural, congenital defects in my feet began leading to endless but often undiagnosed stress fractures. I crazily took a pain killing injection prior to an NBA playoff game one day and the navicular bone in my foot—the centerpiece of the arch—split in half. I have spent the rest of my life chasing the dream of being part of something special and getting back to the top of the mountain one more time.

When I could play ball no more forever, I made the decisive choice to pursue broadcasting as a career despite—or maybe because -being 6'11", having red hair, freckles, a big nose, a goofy nerdy looking face, being a lifelong stutterer unable to speak at all until I was 28 years old, and being a Dead Head having been to now more than 889 Grateful Dead concerts—that television seemed like my obvious next station on the line.

I couldn't get a job in the beginning. They told me repeatedly, "Come on Walton, we're not putting you on TV. You'll get up there and start stuttering and spitting all over everything and everybody; and you'll be quoting Jerry Garcia, Bob Dylan and Neil Young. We simply can't have that!"

After a very slow start in the media business, I was ultimately able to climb into the game and on to the mountain one more time.

18 years after I started broadcasting I was named one of the top 10 pundits in all media, one of the top 20 sports business representatives across the planet and one of the 50 greatest sportscasters of all time.

During that time I never missed an assignment. I signed up and volunteered for everything that I could possibly take on. And more.

Then after countless years of hundreds of nights on the business road every year, with the numbing hundreds of thousands of yearly domestic air miles on and in endlessly bad airplanes, hotels and cars; furniture built for pre-school children; low ceilings and all the disastrous problems and waste, of life on the road, race and run, my spine ultimately collapsed and failed completely.

I spent the next 2 years on the ground. My life was over. I can only describe the unrelenting, excruciating and debilitating pain as being submerged in a vat of scalding acid with an electrifying current running through it, and I could never get out—ever.

What was left of my life was not worth living. If I had a gun, I would have used it. I was standing on the edge of the bridge knowing full well that it was better to jump than to go back to what I had. When you're in that space—it is all so very clear. If you haven't been there—you have no idea.

I had clean-out and reconstructive spine surgery. 8 ½ hours. 4 incisions. Bolts, rods, an erector-set cage to hold it all together, and spacers between the vertebrae. Massive amounts of life-draining and spirit-zapping pain medication. And then the long hard climb back. Into the game of life. Onto the mountain. One more time.

When you go from thinking you're going to die; to wanting to die; to being afraid you're going to live; and then you get better—nothing is really ever the same again.

And when you do finally get better—you can never stop ringing the chimes of freedom.

I'm lucky. I have gotten better. I had no idea what life was like without back pain. Thanks to the discipline, dedication, sacrifice and vision of my spine surgeon, UCSD's Dr. Steve Garfin, and the medical device company that came up with the innovative technology, techniques, procedures and equipment that saved my life, I am now back into the game and onto the mountain one more time.

And while you ultimately learn that health is everything—something that you hear all the time, but never really believe, understand or accept until you don't have it—that is only the beginning.

From there you must have your family or supportive team to carry you through the tough times.

Then you need your home—your sanctuary and safe haven— a place to restore, regroup and recharge for the age old battles that we sometimes won before.

The hope and dream for a better tomorrow is the final piece in your game plan for the trip to the Promised Land.

But these are all really the easy parts. I've been there. More times that I care to remember.

The hard part is getting back to a point and place where you can start the climb—the part where you're still going down in free fall or when you're just wallowing around in the muck of the bottom.

And that is where your core foundation, life skills, and your faith and patience are so severely tested.

When you're on the ground and you can't get up; when the ball has bounced the other way; when no matter what you do you can't seem to get it turned your way, can't find the rhythm, beat or pace, or your way home—the most important factors are—do you still believe, and are you willing to spend the lifetime that it takes to get to where you need and want to be?

Some will claim that it's just about hard work. Nonsense. If it was just about hard work, nobody would ever fail. Hard work is a constant, and anybody who wants to can do that.

Smart, intelligent work. Structure. Discipline. Perseverance. Persistence. Luck. The team. A plan. The dream. That's what you really need—in mega-doses.

Put aside your pride and stubbornness, and let other people help you. They definitely want to, but until you let them in, you have no chance. This fight can't be won alone. And nobody ever makes it to the top alone.

In the early days when all seems lost as you spiral helplessly and hopelessly down, don't fight the tide or rip currents; let it flow, even if it's still downhill. The temptation is to try to make small adjustments on the perimeter and to address minor issues. That won't get it done. And you find yourself fighting the losing battle of beating, short-changing and cheating yourself—the worst kind of defeat you'll ever suffer, the kind you'll never get over.

But the big picture solutions are impossible to see clearly or implement until you've hit the bottom. Once you've cratered, and the turn has been made, the rest is easy, and everything becomes crystal clear.

Always come back to the beginning, to your foundation and core—take a step back and start over—closing the circle of life one more time.

The foundation of your stable health program has to include exercise, water, fresh air and sunshine.

The end of the line—or the beginning, it's really the same thing and place—for all of us in the world and culture of sport and health is the water, the weight room and the bike.

Get in the warm water. Move. Stretch. Dream. All weightless. Get to the places comfortably that you can't possibly reach in the air.

The weight room allows you to develop and minimize the weaknesses and limitations that life causes.

The bike pulls it all together. And all of it without the impact and compression that eventually grinds and crushes us.

My bike is my wheelchair, my gym and my church all in one magnificent package of technology, innovation, comfort and efficiency.

You will get better. Don't give up. You can make it.

You won't believe it at the beginning. But you have to do everything to give yourself the chance. Don't beat yourself. This is all hard enough without you being your own worst enemy.

Accept that the bottom is where you will learn a new concept of "everything".

And when you do get better, as I have, you will not remember how awful it all was. The body, spirit and soul are most remarkable in that after the healing, the pain will truly be gone. All of it.

You have earned and been given the greatest gift of all—a chance to play in the game of life one more day.

But don't wait. Get started. Go your own way. Chase your dream. The finished product is most often a result of incremental progress. Waiting for things to fall totally and completely into place is a self-defeating, excuse-laden, prophetical trap. Chase it down. Get into the game.

When you're on that long hard climb back into the game of life, never forget the people who helped you along the way back and up. The same people who selflessly sacrificed and lived for you—for your chance to play one more day.

And when you do make it home yourself—happy and healthy—don't be the guy who turns around and pulls the ladder up behind him. No. That's not the way life works. Turn around and reach back down with an open and extended hand to help the next guy up and in.

I am the luckiest guy in the world. I have had 37 orthopedic operations. Both of my ankles are fused. My knees, hands and wrists don't work. I have a fused spine. And I just had my knee replaced after dragging that bad, bent, crooked, mangled leg around for the last 49 years.

Other than that, everything is fine.

Strangely, I am a better and happier person today because of all the troubles.

In my bleakest of moments several wonderful friends gave me some powerful and consistent encouragement. Their daily support was invaluable. It was easy to memorize and repeat; nearly impossible to execute.

He who's not busy being born is busy dying.

You can't finish what you don't start.

Let's go! Who wants to come out and play today?

Good luck, health, family and fortune.

Please let me know how I can ever help you.

I'll see you on the climb, and I'll do my best to keep the cheap talk to a minimum.

–Bill Walton

AUTHOR'S NOTE

Medical records are routinely a matter of utmost privacy. The Health Insurance Portability and Accountability Act (HIPAA) sets the standard for sensitive patient data protection. Patient privacy regarding the circumstances of major spine surgery is most certainly subject to the requirements set forth under HIPAA. All of the patients who have shared their experiences in this book have given permission to use their private information in the hope that their experience may help others find their way out of a life of chronic pain.

When the patient contributors read the first draft of this book, one of them asked to have a pseudonym used in the final product. With an abundance of caution, I have removed the surnames of the patients and replaced them with only their last initial. The sole exception is patient Doug Amend, who suggested a brilliant addendum to the book regarding the duties and challenges facing the caregiver. I identify him by his proper name as he is also identified as the author of the addendum.

All of the statements in this book are transcriptions of interviews that I conducted over a six-month period. Although the names of the patients have been altered, the medical professionals who contributed to The Optimized Patient are identified by their professional names and titles.

As orthopedic surgeons became aware of the first draft of this book, they requested that I broaden the scope to include knee, ankle, hip, shoulder, elbow wrist, etc. I have had a partial knee replacement subsequent to my three spine surgeries and I can personally attest to the fact that the optimized approach to preparation and recovery is equally applicable for many other surgeries and major injuries. In this updated edition I have included interviews with surgeons who have a specialty that is other than spine surgery.

1

IT'S A COMMITMENT

When I started thinking about writing this book, "it's a commitment" were the first words that came to mind. When you think about it, you wouldn't be considering, or be scheduled for, major surgery if you weren't *committed* to living a better quality of life. For those of you who may be simply recovering from a serious injury without surgery, please understand that the challenge of major injury recovery is exactly the same. Increasingly, medical professionals, insurance carriers, and medical device companies are working to better inform prospective patients about the path to a healthy life free of pain. *The Optimized Patient* is both a guidebook on how to prepare for and recover from surgery and major injuries and the gateway to a community of people who, like you, have made a commitment to get well and live a pain-free life. Although my personal experience with crippling pain was associated with spine surgery, *The Optimized Patient* is an important resource for anyone and everyone who is considering or scheduled for surgery or recovering from a major injury.

The premise that you are in control of your outcome is the foundation of *The Optimized Patient* concept. Your doctors are going to do their part, but without your help an optimized outcome is uncertain at best. Too many patients forget—or choose to ignore—their role in achieving the pain-free life they are dreaming about. I am not a doctor or a medical practitioner of any kind. I am also not an athlete or particularly physically fit. I also don't possess any special knowledge beyond what I experienced before, during, and after my surgeries. Simply, I have the best possible training and most important credential necessary to write about the patient experience: I was a patient and I recovered. Just like you, I am a person who faced the very serious challenges that are a part of a serious injury and major surgery. But, I made a choice before I committed to surgery to not be just another patient. I made a commitment to be an optimized patient—and you can do it too.

The ironic part of the story is that I didn't even know what an optimized patient was or how to be one until years after my first surgery. There was no book. Common sense told me that six hours of surgery with incisions in my belly, right side, and back were going to knock me down a peg or two, or three. It made sense to me that I needed to prepare—to get as healthy as I could, to get my head on straight, to eat well, to strengthen my core, to prepare my home for the post-operative recovery and mobility challenges. I didn't know it then, but all of that can be summarized in a single word: optimize. For me, becoming optimized consisted of one part research, one part intuition, and two parts dumb luck. I researched what the latest technology and techniques were for my surgery. Luckily, my nephew, who is an anesthesiologist in New

York, suggested I look into procedures other than a laminectomy. Over lunch, an attorney friend of mine gave me a lucky referral for a second opinion. The surgeon who gave me the second opinion told me about a different and emerging approach to spine surgery. In my gut, I knew I had lucked into a better approach. Consider your finding this book part of your dumb luck. What I learned over seven years is now yours in less than five hours of reading. But, like I said, to make it work for you—it's a commitment.

For six months, I built my core strength knowing that all the muscle and nerve damage from the incisions was going to limit my ability to bend, lift, and twist for many weeks. It made sense to me that the stronger I was before surgery, the faster I would be able to regain normal function. I am sure that makes sense to you as well. I made the commitment and struggled in the gym with the pain and discomfort that was part of my back injury to get ready for the big day. It wasn't fun, but it was necessary to optimize. Unfortunately, there was a huge flaw in my recovery plan that nobody was writing about. On my return home, with walker and back brace, the last thing I wanted to do was shop and cook. A month's supply of frozen food seemed like a fair solution. I have learned it was a terrible solution and a fundamental error for an optimized recovery; more about that in Chapter 11. You won't have to make those mistakes because this book curates all the best ideas to use and worst mistakes to avoid before, during, and after surgery.

Living a healthy life is not easy or convenient. It's a commitment. I am going to say that often in this book. In the broadest sense, living an optimized life—with or without surgery—is a commitment. I am writing about the surgical experience because it shines a spotlight on the desperate need for an optimized lifestyle. At no time in your life will the struggle to be optimized be more challenging to attain or reap you greater rewards than when you are on your way to the operating room. Patients who have committed to major surgery do so because they are determined to get better, to stop the pain. It took me seven years as a patient to discover the parts and pieces of the optimized formula. Every painful and healing lesson I learned is in this book.

The Optimized Patient is equally valuable to surgeons who want the best possible outcome for their patients. As we will hear from several surgeons, surgery is just a part of stopping the pain and becoming you again. The rest, the really hard part, is up to you. It's a commitment to giving your body the help it needs to heal fully. It's a commitment to yourself and to your loved ones to be fully you again. **Optimizing for surgery is a commitment whose successful achievement can be the priceless gift of good health.**

On June 24, 2010, a car accident set into motion a series of events in my life that resulted in this book. There is a wonderful ancient Chinese parable about the fortunate farmer that warrants telling here. I think you will find it both amusing and inspiring and very relevant to your own situation. Finding the good in the most tragic and unfortunate moments in your life is part of the mindset needed to be an optimized patient. Enjoy the story . . .

An old farmer was working in his field with his old sick horse. The farmer felt compassion for the horse and desired to lift its burden. So, he let his horse loose to go the mountains and live out the rest of its life.

Soon after, neighbors from the nearby village visited, offering their condolences and said, "What a shame. Now your only horse is gone. How unfortunate you are! You must be very sad. How will you live, work the land, and prosper?"

The farmer replied: "Who knows? We shall see."

Two days later the old horse came back now rejuvenated after meandering in the mountainsides while eating the wild grasses. He came back with twelve new younger and healthy horses which followed the old horse into the corral. Word got out in the village of the old farmer's good fortune and it wasn't long before people stopped by to congratulate the farmer on his good luck.

"How fortunate you are!" they exclaimed. "You must be very happy!"

Again, the farmer softly said, "Who knows? We shall see."

The next morning, the farmer's only son set off to attempt to train the new wild horses, but the farmer's son was thrown to the ground and broke his leg. One by one villagers arrived during the day to bemoan the farmer's latest misfortune. "Oh, what a tragedy! Your son won't be able to help you farm with a broken leg. You'll have to do all the work yourself, how will you survive? You must be very sad," they said.

Calmly going about his usual business the farmer answered, "Who knows? We shall see."

Several days later a war broke out. The Emperor's men arrived in the village demanding that young men come with them to be conscripted into the Emperor's army. As it happened, the farmer's son was deemed unfit because of his broken leg. "What very good fortune you have!!" the villagers exclaimed as their own young sons were marched away. "You must be very happy."

"Who knows? We shall see!" replied the old farmer as he headed off to work his field alone.

As time went on the broken leg healed but the son was left with a slight limp. Again, the neighbors came to pay their condolences. "Oh, what bad luck. Too bad for you!"

But the old farmer simply replied; "Who knows? We shall see."

As it turned out the other young village boys had died in the war and the old farmer and his son were the only able-bodied men capable of working the village lands. The old farmer became wealthy and was very generous to the villagers. They said: "Oh how fortunate we are, you must be very happy."

To which the old farmer replied, "Who knows? We shall see!"

The damage to my lumbar spine, although not apparent for three days, nearly crippled me on the fourth day. And oddly in line with this story, it left me with a limp. Years of excruciating pain led to the surgeon's office where I considered the need for spine surgery—a frightening idea for any sober person. But, the good news is ten years later my journey to recover from a tragic accident has given me the credentials to help millions of people to optimize and become whole again. Yes, we shall see.

The "*if I can do this, you can do this*" strategy laid out in this book is part of the mental conditioning intended to prepare you for surgery and to help you to recover as fully and rapidly as possible. Targeted nutrition, a positive mental attitude, restorative activity and healing rest are the pillars of creating an optimized patient ready for the challenge of surgery. Over the course of ten years I've been fortunate to meet and to benefit from skilled surgeons, trainers, and nutritional strategists who have helped create the opportunity for my body to do what it was intended to do—to heal itself.

In recent years, the reliance on medication to combat disease has yielded to a more balanced and informed approach where many diseases such as diabetes, hypertension, and high cholesterol have been managed by modifications to nutrition and physical activity. Pharmaceutical management has become unnecessary in many cases. Becoming an "optimized patient," one who has learned from the successful strategies of patients who have gone before, can help you to prepare for, survive, and recover in an optimal way. In our strategy, the optimal way relies more on good thinking, great nutrition, appropriate physical activity and quality rest than it does on pharmaceutical intervention. Learn more about this in Chapter 7.

But let me caution you, if you are looking for a book that says Western medicine is bad or doesn't work, this is not a book for you. Western medicine has developed countless lifesaving drugs. You need only watch television for a couple of hours to see the incredible array of medications that are curing illness, relieving pain, and saving lives. But, you will also note that many of those drugs have side effects that are part of the necessary evil of the good they do. We believe that there are many approaches and methods employed by Western medicine that are essential for healing, but that they often have the side effects of leaving the body in a state of "dis-ease." This is especially true, if not glaringly obvious, in the surgical scenario. Surgery has several side effects to it that merit some common sense and serious consideration.. Read more about that in Chapter 11.

Let's think about a broken arm in a cast. Is the cast healing your arm? Well, no, your arm is healing your arm; the cast is just helping what is natural and engineered into your body to happen.

Your body knows what to do. If that's true, and it is, the cast is just an aid to help the healing along. What we propose here is an optimized strategy that, like the cast for a broken bone, will **allow your body to do what it was meant to do, heal itself.**

It is interesting, and liberating, to write this book from the standpoint of a patient, not a doctor. As you will see, this is not a book about research and graphs and data and pie charts. It is a book about the patient experience. Six patients who have suffered with chronic and debilitating back pain discuss our challenges and the considerations that went into deciding to put our lives in the hands of our surgeons. Several of us had degenerative joint problems while others had a serious accident. I had both. In Chapters 3 and 4, I share what happened to each of us and what we did about it. Read those stories carefully. Whether you fell on a basketball court like Bill Walton or fell off a mountain like financial advisor, Doug Amend, I believe you will find your fears and your own hopes in our heartfelt sharing of what happened to us. By the time you finish this book you will realize that if we could do it, you can too.

None of us knows when we are going to get sick. But, we do know when we're going to have surgery; the exception being, of course, emergency surgery. Many surgeries are scheduled weeks if not months in advance. In my particular case I had six months to prepare for my surgery. I made every day count to add strength to my core and increase my stamina. I knew that in six months I was going to be "hit by a bus." In my surgical experience I was given anesthesia, flushed with antibiotics, and then given opioids to control pain. The outcome was serious constipation that was remedied by stool softeners and a variety of other drugs. When you consider the incisions and the hardware and the stitches and staples, "hit by a bus" is right on the money. My body's natural need upon awakening was to fill it full of the best nutrition that money could buy to aid the healing process. That's plain common sense. The problem was, after anesthesia, antibiotics, and opioids, no matter how good the food was, it couldn't be processed and absorbed by my body with maximum efficiency. I'm going to go way out on a limb and say that almost every surgical patient, or patient recovering from a major injury, has a similar experience: you will be gassed, flushed with antibiotics, and given opioids to control pain. The outcome is the same in almost every patient—a paralyzed and constipated digestive tract that is unable to function well and unable to fully absorb the nutrients necessary for healing. It was a major event three days later when I was able to pass gas! That was the signal that my intestines had "woken up."

This brings to mind the change in operative procedures from decades ago where patients were left in bed for days post-surgery. Despite the fact that I had two lumbar fusions with incisions in my belly, back, and right side, the doctors had me on my feet within an hour of me waking up. What we are suggesting here is a similar approach to the postoperative scenario regarding recovery of digestive performance needed to quickly and fully heal. You will need to wake up and optimize your gut and I will share with you in Chapter 11 what I learned by painful trial and error.

The surgical patient experience is one of those very complex subjects where vital information is fragmented and scattered among a variety of disciplines. I was fortunate to have been treated by gifted surgeons and skilled rehabilitation specialists who gave me the inspiration and insight needed to write a comprehensive plan to both prepare for surgery and fully recover in rehab. Along the way, I was able to heal sufficiently to stop taking all the prescription drugs that had been part of my life for many years. The injury to my spine caused a neurogenic bladder. Simply put, like the neurological issues that caused me to limp, my bladder muscles weren't getting a strong enough signal from my brain to fully contract. The solution was four years of self-catheterization six times a day. If you just winced, you got it right. On top of that I was taking Tamsulosin and Bethanacol to shrink my prostate and stimulate my bladder. Unrelated to my lumbar problems, I was also taking statins for cholesterol. After three months of optimizing I lost 21 pounds and was allowed to stop taking all of those drugs after being examined by my doctors. The natural outcome of a healthy state is a reduced need for medications. Part of what we will explore in Chapter 11 is a nutritional strategy to let food work in conjunction with medicine to fuel your recovery. This is not a revolutionary idea from the contributors to this book. Rather, this is a centuries-old understanding voiced by Hippocrates himself: **"Let food be thy medicine and medicine be thy food."**

People don't normally do things if they don't make sense to them. The notable exception, of course, is religion; believers just believe. To the believers who read this book, you already believe that what you eat and how you move can radically change your life for the better. The experiences of patients recounted in the chapters ahead are intended, for both thinkers and believers, to deliver you into a mind-set that will help you succeed at achieving an improved quality of life. The thinkers and fact-oriented people reading this book may find comfort in the comments from medical professionals and therapists. To be clear, *The Optimized Patient* is not a research project—it's a handbook. Like the story of the fortunate farmer, sometimes luck plays as significant a role as science in achieving the desired outcome.

Another part of the dumb luck aspect of my becoming an optimized patient was meeting NBA Hall of Fame basketball star Bill Walton. Bill had the same kind of spine surgery that I had. I met him at a gathering of spine patients, some of whom I quote in this book. Bill immediately engaged and coached me—urged me—to get into a swimming pool every day. I thought I was doing great work on my rehab, but Bill woke me up to what it takes to really recover. It takes a lot of work, and someone to guide you, which will be addressed in Chapter 9. What you will learn is that optimizing is one of those ideas that is simple, but not easy. I don't know about you, but I have seen so many social media videos that promise to give you the secret to great health if you will only watch their 30-minute educational video. It usually ends with a doctor or some authority selling you their pill or powder or potion that will make it all better. *The Optimized Patient* is not about selling you another supplement like those social media films. If anything, **we are going to teach you how to properly use your grocery store to support what your body is programmed to do—heal.**

The Optimized Patient has a four "pillars" understanding of what it takes to meet your challenge head on in surgery and get better: a positive mental attitude, quality rest, fresh food, and therapeutic exercise. The first of the four, mindset or positive mental attitude, is where the way back to your best self begins. Without a positive mental attitude, the other three essential pillars will be a burden rather than an exciting opportunity to get better and live a fuller life.. The "will to be well", as you will learn from several surgeons in Chapter 6 and 10, is the fundamental ingredient to a full recovery and a return to normal function. It all begins with believing in you.

If you are injured, suffering from a chronic condition or planning major surgery, you understand challenges in your life. Whether it's the challenge of getting through the day without pain pills, finding a comfortable position so you can sleep through the night, walking around the grocery store, or standing at the stove, we are all facing the daily challenge of chronic pain and the inability to live full and pain-free lives. That was the real challenge: not living my life fully. Everyone who has made the commitment to prepare for and recover from surgery has found it challenging, very challenging. You will too. Likewise, every one of those patients who committed to optimize traded a temporary and painful challenge of surgery or the hard work of recovery for the lifelong benefit of a healthier life, free of the painful misery that tainted every aspect of their lives before. **To achieve your pain-free goal you have to have the will to be well.** It is the first part of the commitment.

So, let's talk about the gap between what you think your body will do and what your "will" can help you to achieve. Mack Newton is a renowned physical trainer and teacher. Not long after my car accident, I was fortunate to participate in one of his exercise classes. Like many of the genuine yoga studios, Mack keeps his "dojo" at a toasty 100 degrees or more. Many of his regulars are professional athletes. Mack taught me that "your will can carry you when your body fails you." I thought he was crazy—until I experienced it personally. When your body says "stop!" your will can give you the power to carry on. This is not to say or to recommend that your activity should further injure your body by overdoing it. However, I learned that I had more capacity to do the necessary work to get better than my mind believed and my body would allow. I just needed the will to do it. Becoming an optimized patient relies on that exact mindset. You need the will to go to physical therapy to get the needed education and conditioning. You need the will to get well to get you to the grocery store, so you can prepare fresh food that will help your body to heal.

From chiropractors to epidurals, I tried everything to put a stop to the pain in my legs. I knew I had "compression" in my lower back. I knew it was serious. I knew there were surgical options. I also knew that there were too many horror stories online about surgeries that went wrong. From people with rods in their back who were actually paralyzed for life to amputees who had their good leg removed instead of the bad, I read about too many surgeries that had gone horribly wrong. You cannot possibly be in your right mind if those stories do not give you pause when considering major surgery. Personally, I was afraid of going down the surgical road because I was making a decision today on information from yesterday. Medicine and surgical technique and technology are evolving at an increasingly rapid pace. The surgeons address the horror stories of the past in Chapter 5. As a patient, I made it my business to do my homework. Increasingly, the doctors who perform spine surgery and the medical device companies who make the hardware necessary to accomplish effective spinal fusion, have realized that a patient's understanding of the reality of spinal fusion is quite different *after* the surgery. Let me illustrate with my own experience, since I did it three times. This fear-based reluctance to get after your best outcome is also prevalent in people who are recovering from major injuries with or without surgery.

My fear-ridden psychological "mindset" for the first surgery differed vastly from my confidence going into the second surgery. It was Mark Twain who famously said, "Some of the worst things in my life never even happened." All of the very frightening things that I had heard about spine surgery were rattling around in my head. And just like Mark Twain, the worst of it never happened. As I prepared for my second spine surgery, I had none of the fears or concerns that gripped me the first time. I felt compelled to share this realization with my spine surgeon. I told him I was contemplating writing about my experiences and he helped facilitate connecting me with the other patients who also generously share their very personal medical experiences in this book.

It's a big decision to put your spine and your life in the hands of a surgeon. It's a little awkward to ask a surgeon, "Hey, have you killed or crippled anyone?" As a joke, I once asked my cardiologist if any of his patients had ever died, knowing that sooner or later they *all* do. We had a good laugh over that and I have been in his care as my internist for the last 30 years. Unless your doctor takes himself way too seriously, it's acceptable to ask your doctor tough questions. The stakes are very high and your questions should be many and bluntly probing. We will take a close look at that in Chapter 8.

Even though I asked those questions of my doctor directly, that did not address *my* risk and all of the horror stories I had heard about back surgery. Remember I said that dumb luck often plays into your best outcome? Just prior to scheduling my date for surgery I had lunch with an attorney friend of mine. During lunch he revealed to me that he had just had back surgery. The exact L2/3 and L4/5 fusion that I was considering (the "L" indicates lumbar and the number indicates location). Finally, someone to talk to about all the question marks surrounding my choice of surgeons and procedures! And now you have a book that will give you critically important answers and insights too.

The Optimized Patient was researched and written to answer the most frequently asked question, "Is it worth the risk to do this and can I be myself again?" Can I fully recover? If you decide that your particular problem and the exact solution that you are considering is worth the risk, the next question you ask should be, "How do I prepare to get the best possible results?" If you are thinking, "Shouldn't my doctor be able to answer that question?" Yes, your doctor should be. However, there is a management saying that suggests "nobody knows everything, but everybody knows something." Again, I am writing from my personal experience with a surgeon who is among the best in the world, performing the latest and greatest in advanced procedures. You will hear directly from him and two other surgeons in Chapter 6. But, pre-operative conditioning, both with physical therapy and targeted nutrition, is not a surgeon's area of expertise. Likewise, post-operative strategies, including the psychological importance of a positive mindset are not their field either. It is impossible for me to overstate my surgeon's personal excitement about my writing this book so his patients could learn about all the pillars of the optimized process.

The bottom line: if you are not asking questions about pre-operative conditioning and post-operative recovery/healing strategies, you should be. I had no one to ask. Luckily, I had the benefit of many years of yoga practice, bicycling, and gym membership. Although my activity was diminished after my car accident, I knew the fundamentals of how to get into shape. Not everyone is fortunate to be in reasonably good health prior to surgery. I just knew intuitively that on December 22nd I was going to "get hit by a bus." Knowing that I was going to have a seriously traumatic experience in the operating room, it only made sense to brace myself by getting into the best possible physical condition. I have no doubt it makes sense to you too. But, how do you do it in a way that is right for you? Who can you ask?

As I will explain in the following chapter, you are not alone. If you don't have a friend who has had spine surgery or recovered from a major trauma, or if you can't find or don't have a support group anywhere in your community, you have in your hand the next best thing. Together with the website at www.TheOptimizedPatient.com you have the tools you need to help your body do what it was designed and programmed to do—heal itself. It's a mental as well as a physical challenge. If you have the will to be well and have access to a community of people who have done what you are about to do, it's a commitment you can manage—and you are not alone.

2

YOU ARE NOT ALONE

Imagine that you are at a dinner party and six people who have successfully recovered from major spine surgery are gathered at a large table. Then, three spine surgeons, two orthopedic surgeons, two physical therapists, and a chiropractor sit down to join them in a discussion about how to optimize for spine surgery. To top it off, a PhD who is a Registered Dietician Nutritionist (RDN) shows up to share how food plays a major role in optimizing for and recovering from surgery. Now imagine that they are gathered at the table just to help *you* understand if surgery is right for you. Well, that's exactly where you're sitting and exactly what we hope to do. In the time it takes to read this book, those patients, surgeons, and experts are going to share their experiences and knowledge to give you the information you need to make a confident and well-informed decision about whether or not spine surgery is right for you. And should you make that decision, you will have the best information possible to achieve what every spine patient wants: to be you again. Whether you are scheduled for spine surgery or recovering from a fall off a scissor-lift, the recovery process is exactly the same.

Before I introduce you to the patients, I would like to share with you why having a team to coach you through the challenge of spine surgery and injury recovery is so important. Every year on January 1st legions of people make their New Year's resolution to go to the gym. They put down their money and make the commitment to do whatever it takes to drop those holiday pounds and live a healthier lifestyle. By the middle of January most of them have forgotten that commitment and have returned to the bad habits that ruined their health in the first place. But, some do commit and make it stick. In particular, people who have a trainer, a coach, or a workout buddy. The "If he can do it, I can do it" mindset is a super powerful motivator. Accountability to a set of goals makes sure you will stay on track. Coaches report that many of their most successful clients began in a place of fear and doubt. I am going to share with you the experiences and thoughts of several spine patients who overcame their fear and doubt, made the commitment, and achieved their goals of a better quality of life. Our patients want you to know that it really is true: if they can do it, you can do it. What we want you to know is that you don't have to do it alone—and you shouldn't!

My personal journey led me to understand that reliable information and genuine shared experiences are critical to your full recovery. Just like the newbies on January 1st at the gym, you need the right mindset too. You likely already have the will to get well or you wouldn't be reading this book. This chapter is about getting to know the community of people who have put behind them what lies ahead for you. The first step to becoming an optimized patient is sourcing the best available information about how to prepare for, survive, and fully recover from surgery or a major injury. Where better to source that information than from the patients themselves? As you read the thoughts and experiences of the contributors we have assembled to advise you, keep repeating to yourself, **"If they can do it, I can do it."**

Every spine patient has a story. Most of those stories are truly remarkable. Consider the story of Doug Amend. He fell off a mountain. Really, he fell off a mountain and lived. The amazing part of his story is that falling 300 feet wasn't the worst part of it. The really amazing part is the eight-hour ordeal that he endured dragging himself out of the wilderness to get help—with a broken back. True to the premise of this book, I felt that my car crash wasn't all that bad compared to what he went through. After reading this you may not feel that what you're going through is so bad after all, either. That "feeling" is the beginning the mindset needed for a full recovery.

Having fallen off the mountain, believing his ribs were broken, Doug called Search and Rescue. This is where Doug's story begins in his own words. He will tell his full story in Chapter 3.

> Search and rescue says, "You have to have a life-threatening injury or be incapacitated. You're not. Do you have a first aid kit?"
>
> I said, "Yes, I do."
>
> Search and Rescue says, "Well, look in it for Ibuprofen. I'd take a couple of those to help with the rib pain and, you know, start hiking."

> It took me eight hours. So, when I got in the emergency room, the doctor assessed me saying, "Well, there's nothing we really can do for broken ribs. Your arms are black and blue. You've got a nice road rash on your left cheek. We'll go ahead and order an X-ray as a precaution. Okay. Well, we got some bad news. You didn't break any ribs, but you broke your back."
>
> It was the T11 vertebrae in a burst fracture.

Yes, Doug hiked eight hours out of the wilderness with a broken back.

If you are shaking your head in disbelief, that makes two of us.

Linda B. is a homemaker. She didn't fall off a mountain, survive a car crash, or have any trauma at all. Yet, she was suffering from excruciating back pain and tried every conceivable remedy possible. None of what was happening to Linda made any sense. She recalls how her problems started.

> So, after I had my second child, I started having back issues. And at the time I was in North Carolina. So, we went to the head of Duke University Sports Medicine, so this guy had credentials. I went for a consultation with him, and he said, "Wow, you have severe degenerative disc disease, which is unusual for your age." At that time I think I was 37. And he said, "You would benefit from a spinal fusion."
>
> And that was the first I had ever heard of it. So, I got a second opinion. And I don't recall if the leg pain started then? I think it did. Yeah, because that's one of

> the indicators of whether they can help you or not, and of how severe you are. But most of what I remember is the back pain. So, I got the second opinion; they said the same thing. And at that time, I had a brand-new baby and a toddler. And it was the first time I had heard the words back surgery. And so, I did every single modality in the book. Well not every single one, but I tried quite a few different ones. Chiropractic helped me along the way. Oh, and I remember, I got my first steroid shot; it was such a simple thing. He said, "Oh, I can give you a steroid shot," and I lifted up my shirt, bent over, and he gave me an easy shot in the back. And that helped for years. That got me through quite a few years. Along with chiropractic, stretching, and exercise . . . what else did I do? Ibuprofen, not all the time, though, because if you keep using that it doesn't work anymore either.

Homemaker Linda B. discovered she had early onset degenerative disc disease after her second child.

Linda's experience was common to all of the patients who are quoted in this book. There is a natural aversion to going straight out to see the spine surgeon or committing to any major surgery. As the title of this chapter suggests, you are not alone in your experience. In Chapter 4, "What Are My Options?" we will take a closer look at what the patients tried and what worked—and what didn't. There actually is a method for determining if you really need a surgeon or not.

Sometimes spine issues and many workplace injuries develop in an instant from a trauma. Sometimes spine issues develop over time. Sometimes it is both. Consider the case of recent retiree, Robert G.

> I actually turned 55 today. Well, my back problems started probably about 20 years ago, in my mid-30s. I just retired from Bridgestone/Firestone, so I've been in the retail business for 30 years and on my feet, running an automotive shop. And, I think part of that had to do with this, constantly being on my feet 10 to 12 hours a day.
>
> Some of it was degenerative disc disease, but it all originally started one night when I sneezed in the middle of the night and my back just locked up and I literally could not get out of bed. I think it took me about 45 minutes to crawl from the bed to the restroom that morning. I was in such pain that I just stayed in bed and took Advil and pain relievers for about five to six days before I could get out and even get into a vehicle to go to a doctor. Once I was able to get to the doctor, they did the MRIs, did x-rays, did everything and said that it definitely looked like I had issues with my disc. I can't remember exactly everything they had said, but degenerative disc disease was part of it. They gave me a cortisone shot.
>
> At the time I was quite physically fit. I was in martial arts and so exercising daily, stretching daily. I was in probably one of the best times of fitness in my life. And,

> it literally started all from that. I mean, obviously something was going on because I don't think just a sneeze would cause that to happen. I think a lot of it had to do with just my occupation, being on my feet all the time, constantly on concrete floors definitely, definitely took its toll over some time.

Robert G., after years of undiagnosed degenerative disc disease, was incapacitated by a sneeze!

We usually think of back problems as beginning in our 40s. Certainly, that is the demographic that the makers of over-the-counter pain relievers seem to think based on the actors they feature in those ads. But, Joy H. started having neck pain when she was a child. Everyone thought it was because of the hours she dedicated to her very serious violin practice. Perhaps Joy's story is like yours. Joy remembered,

> It began when I was 11 years old. I started playing the violin at that time. That is the reason we missed it. We missed all the signals. I knew I was having pain, but we associated it with the violin playing. My back hurt, usually only when I practiced my violin, and it would go away after. Sometimes it would linger if I practiced more and more, as I grew into the profession. Sometimes it would still be there in the evening, and my mom would rub my back. I never really thought much about it, it just kinda crept up. It got gradually worse, until about the time I was 18.

> I had just finished high school, I was teaching the violin and playing and performing full-time. One day I had had a particularly long day, nine hours of teaching and playing. I got in my car to drive home, and the pain . . . I guess it just penetrated through my thoughts, and I realized "I'm in chronic pain." I didn't notice. It kind of got me all of a sudden. I think as a kid, you just do what you've got to do to make it through, and I hadn't really stopped to consider what normal was like. I was really afraid. I had a hard time moving my arms to drive myself home. I was afraid I wouldn't be able to drive myself home. Sheer willpower got me through that car ride. I talked to my parents. I said, "Okay, we need to see somebody. This is really serious, and my friends aren't going through this. I guess it's not normal."

Joy H., a young violinist, learned that the agony she was feeling in her arms from a degenerating disc had nothing to do with hours of practice and teaching.

If Lucio D. is anything, he is a people person. As talkative as he is likable, his trouble started when he was rear-ended in a near fatal car crash. He faced many challenges as you will shortly read in his own words. The most interesting part, covered later in the book, is that his injuries prevented him from tilting his head back and looking at the sky. Through all the pain and suffering, his deepest worry was that he would not be able to do the simple thing of just tipping his head back to see the sky. His fear almost prevented him from optimizing his outcome. Lucio D. in his own words,

I am 45 years old. I live in Escondido, California. I'm an entrepreneur-business owner; I open up restaurants and cafes and bars as a family business. Born into it. My parents have been in that business since 1962, and my mom worked pregnant with me at a bar they owned in Germany, so that's how long I was in that business.

I was a very healthy individual, very much in shape. Always worked out, always stayed at the top of my game, and I stopped at a light on the [Interstate] 5 in Cannon Drive, in Carlsbad. I'd just gotten a gig of writing a critic blog for a San Diego website for restaurants and entertainment, so I went around tasting food, watching venues. That was my first day on the job, and then boom, out of the nowhere. Rear-ended at 40 miles per hour. And that's when all my back problems began. That was 2015.

So, I went from being extremely healthy, you know, a guy who could grab a surfboard and go surfing for hours, to barely being able to go to the bathroom. That's how awful it was. Woke up with the paramedic checking my pulse on my neck, because it knocked me out. And my seat actually broke. She hit me so hard that the backboard of the seat snapped in two. But when I came to, there was a lot of pain immediately. I couldn't feel my legs. I felt like my back was broken. I couldn't move my left arm—it had totally gone numb. I was taken to the hospital, and put in traction right in hospital, so I wouldn't move. And they prodded away. They gave me muscle relaxers to make the shock from being hit so hard come down. And then they told me what the injuries were. The abdomen, my cervical vertebrae, C-5, was totally crushed, completely down to paper thin. And the injury to my C-5 was also choking off my spinal cord right there at my neck. So, I wasn't getting much feeling going on to the rest of my body. Both my hands were continuously falling asleep from it. And then I was told that my lumbar 7 disc had been crushed and was protruding and pushing those nerves as well.

After being shattered in a car accident, restaurateur turned journalist, Lucio D., worried if he would ever be himself again. Specifically, would he ever be able to tilt his head back and look up at the sky?

As I mentioned earlier, I was a passenger in a car crash. If ever there was an accident, this crash was a total accident. Like me, Doug's spine challenge began with a trauma. Ironically, it is almost nine years to the day after the accident that this book will be published. I was a passenger in a car at the beginning of a business trip to Evanston, Wyoming. Like many of you reading this book, I suffered a work-related injury. My colleague, Gary, failed to see the stop sign at the end of the off-ramp on Interstate 80. We were hit broad side on the driver's side. The force of the impact totally destroyed the car, spinning it around the intersection. Gary and I eased out of the smoking car, checking each other for blood and broken bones. Miraculously there were none. I had a bruise across my chest from the seatbelt, but other than that, we seemed to be uninjured. What I did not know was that my lumbar spine was silently swelling from the impact. Three days later, at a convention in Las Vegas, I was unable to get out of bed and could not walk.

Every patient believes that no one can really understand what they are going through. The fact is, everyone who contributed to this book all understand exactly what you are going through. We want you to be comforted by the fact that you are not alone in your pain—we have been there and done that. We understand. I asked my surgeon, Dr. Sanjay Khurana, to sum up what had happened to me. I share it here because it helps to underline how badly I was injured and the level of my pain. The only important part of knowing these facts and knowing I recovered is "if I can do, you can do it too!"

Dr. Khurana put it this way:

> The clinical symptoms you came in with were what I call claudication, which is a difficulty walking or standing, atrophy, and dysfunction of the lower extremities. It was also coupled with a condition that may or may not have been related to the accident, a urinary problem, but that wasn't the reason you came for the spinal consultation. When we looked at your imaging, I was struck by how profound the degeneration in your back was at the levels causing the problem. So, really what was going on, was that at your L4/5 level, you had something, not a super uncommon condition, called a Degenerative Spondylolisthesis, which was where you had, basically, a translated disc of L4, a translating L4 upon L5 [please note that this convention L4/5 indicates the two involved bones and the location of the

disc between them]. But that in and of itself wasn't the problem. The major problem was that you had just extraordinary stenosis. In other words, nerve compression at both that level, as well at a separate level, L2/3, which was two levels above that level separated by, what was at that point, a normal level of L3/4. So you had two constriction points: L4/5 had an associated level of instability, and L2/3 had a collapsed disc with a little bit of the scoliosis.

I had leg pain that was so severe that I could not walk. I was a neuron away from spending the rest of my life in a wheelchair.

My special position in the spectrum of spine ailments among the six of us is that I had fusion surgery twice and, sometime later, I had a discectomy. It would seem that three times is a charm and somewhat not the norm. One and done is the goal. Three times is an extraordinary amount of surgery. Although it is by no means a world record, it is significant. You may have noted that the title of this chapter is "You Are Not Alone." It is very common for patients facing major surgery to feel isolated, confused, and alone. The experts introduced in this chapter, a hiker, a homemaker, a sky watcher, a violinist, a retiree, and me—a writer, all experienced some version of what you're going through. I wanted you to meet us and get to know us and what we went through so that you will never feel like you are isolated. Each of us had a very different experience but a very similar outcome. With any luck, the successful pain-free outcome that we all are so grateful for will be yours as well.

I hope you will agree that it is helpful to hear in depth the details of what happened to each of the patients who have contributed to this book. In my interviews with them it was extremely interesting to me to hear not just what happened, but how they struggled to avoid the surgeon. Although understandable, and maybe even prudent, it prolonged the suffering and put a full recovery in jeopardy for each and every one of us.

This is a critical point and really gets to the heart of this book. I avoided seeing a spine doctor for four years. Robert G. struggled with his back pain for 20 years before his situation forced him into the doctor's office. My point isn't that everyone with a back pain, chronic pain or workplace injury should be immediately dialing up the nearest surgeon. On the other hand, there is a point at which not calling the doctor prolongs your pain and degrades your quality of life. As you will learn when we take a deeper look in the next chapter, one of our patient contributors actually considered suicide. Her quality of life was so compromised and her pain so acute that she actually considered whether or not being alive was worth it! When I write that "You Are Not Alone," it is a meaningful and genuine statement. No matter where you are on the hopeful to hopeless spectrum, you will find relevant insight here that may have direct bearing on your mindset.

You will read in Chapter 6, "The Surgeon's Perspective," that there is a real difference between nerve pain and back pain. One needs surgery, the other may not. Most of the horror stories we have either heard about or read about on the Internet are a result of back surgeries that weren't necessary. As you will hear from the doctors themselves, surgeries are often performed that either cure nothing or make the pain worse. Let's meet the surgeons who have joined us at the table.

Dr. Branko Skovrlj is a young, up-and-coming spine surgeon in Wayne, New Jersey. I asked Dr. Branko (because of the rather complex Croatian spelling of his last name, he prefers to be referred to as Dr. Branko) what's most important when a patient is looking for a spine surgeon. He was quick and definite in his answer:

> When I'm talking to the patient, I'm trying to think of being the patient myself so I can help him or her understand what's going on. I think one important thing for the patient is to listen. This is my opinion. You don't have to have surgery with me. You have to have surgery with somebody, somebody who you're first, comfortable with, and second, who, whatever they told you, makes sense to you. But the most important thing is, the patient has to go to somebody who's going to sit down, look them in the eye, and spend more than fifteen, twenty minutes (definitely more than five minutes) before they tell them they need surgery.

Dr. Justin Saliman is the founder and CEO of OutcomeMD and operates out of Cedars-Sinai Hospital in Los Angeles. His surgical specialty is minimally invasive repairs for shoulder, hip and knee. OutomeMD is an application specifically designed to give patients real data on how well patients fared in a doctor's care. Dr. Saliman is concerned about how patients research doctors:

> "Basically, we focus on patient catering instead of patient care in America. The reason is that patients don't have anything else to go by to figure out who's a good

> doctor and who's not a good doctor. There are inadequate resources in existence today for patients to know which doctor to select. In fact, there have been very good studies, like one in the archives of *Internal Medicine*, called "The Cost of Satisfaction," and the sample size was 52,000, so it was a very powerful study. And they found that with five-star doctors, you're more likely to die. There's an inverse relationship between subjective reviews and outcomes. The doctors who are focused on marketing and positioning themselves as a five-star doctor, are less focused on delivering good care.

Dr. Christopher Hills practices in Jackson, Wyoming, at Teton Orthopedics. He was focused on the patient's expectations. Like Dr. Branko, he was very clear about what's most important for a patient in their first conversation with a surgeon.

> You have to take it separately and individually. Point in fact; I live in Jackson Hole, Wyoming, where I treat a much different population than those I treated when I was in spine training in North Carolina. It's not uncommon that I'm seeing a 70 to 80 year old who wants to ski 30 to 60 days a year on the mountain, snow skiing, and they have a spine condition! Their goal is to maintain that lifestyle and continue to ski 30 to 60 days, and so we have to have a heart-to-heart discussion on whether the surgery is going to be able to keep the ability for them to do that.

In Chapter 5, "Accepting the Surgical Fix," I will talk about how each of us as patients came to accept the fact that we had mechanical problems in our backs that could only be fixed by a surgeon. So, what is your role, as the patient, in determining if surgery will be a good thing or bad thing for you? Surprisingly, there is a simple protocol for determining if you need—or don't need—spine surgery. I will detail it in Chapter 4, "What Are My Options?"

I mentioned at the beginning of this chapter that we have a couple of highly trained and effective physical therapists at the table for you to meet. By the way, the time to meet your physical therapist is *before* your surgery. Patti Sogaard, MPT, and Solomon Joseph are two of the physical therapists who lead the team at Advanced Orthopedic Physical Therapy in Signal Hill, California. Patti is the owner and has worked extensively with recovering spine patients. Both of these therapists shared with me the proper role of a physical therapist. I was fortunate to participate in Solomon Joseph's aqua therapy class and he will share with you prehab and rehab strategies that all physical therapists know, but—I believe—few employ because a swimming pool is required to benefit from it. The incredible part of what Solomon recommends is that many patients who follow his protocol find out that they don't need surgery at all.

I asked Patti Sogaard where physical therapy fits into the team of people gathering at the table to give you the information you need to effectively prepare for, survive, and recover from spine surgery. Patti was very emphatic about the critical role of physical therapy in prehab. Patti said, "I usually do not see spine patients for prehab, I will see patients who will rehab to try to avoid surgery, rather than prehab if it's the spine. I usually see patients for prehab if it's say a joint injury such as a knee injury that has increased inflammation and decreased range of motion. So, an MD refers a patient for prehab if there's a traumatic injury, causing swelling or decreased joint function in mobility. Studies have shown if a patient goes into surgery with close to a healthy joint, as close as possible, then recovery afterwards is easier and more likely to be successful. Plus, prehab also gives the patient some education on post-surgical recovery, such as what to expect, and, if they are using an assisted device, how to use it before they go in rather than afterwards. Prehab can not only decrease pain and stiffness before going into surgery, but it can also educate the patient on what to expect after surgery."

Like my aqua therapy coach, Solomon Joseph, Bill Walton is a powerful advocate for aqua therapy. In fact, it was Bill Walton who first told me to get into the pool as part of my recovery. It would make sense that a professional athlete in the Basketball Hall of Fame would know how to recover from injuries! But, you don't need to be a professional athlete to benefit from what professional athletes know and what they do to recover from the injuries that are an occupational hazard. What is the single factor that is most determinative of a good or a bad outcome? A top-notch surgeon? A great hospital? Exceptional nursing? Yes, all of that is really important. But, surprise, *the single most important factor is you.* Remember, the first words of this book: It's a commitment. Many of the worst outcomes from spine surgery were the results of the patient's failure to participate in their own recovery. The surgeons will discuss this in depth as they have observed this phenomenon over years of practice. When I write that you are not alone, that extends beyond the patient and medical community gathered at the table for you. You are also not alone, or on your own, trying to learn how to manage the often frightening and confusing information flow and decision-making process as you consider surgery. Whenever I have had the privilege of talking with a group of spine patients, at some point the question comes up, "What happened to you?" You may find that what is happening to you, happened in some form or another to all of us. You really are not alone.

3

WHAT HAPPENED?

We all come to sit in the doctor's office for the same reason: we hurt and have lost our quality of life. In the case of an accident or workplace injury you have probably come on gurney with red lights flashing. How we got to the place of chronic pain or serious trauma runs the gamut from falling off a mountain to falling on a basketball court to simply doing too much and wearing yourself out. You have already met the five other patients besides me. Now, let's dig more deeply into their stories. I'm pretty sure you will find yourself saying, "Yeah, that's what happened to me." I know that's what I was thinking when I interviewed them. There's a seventh patient who I am saving until the end of the book. He is a screenwriter friend of mine named Adam Rodman. Adam did not have spine surgery, but he did follow *The Optimized Patient* strategy. His surgery was to correct damage done to his septum and sinuses when he was a young man. Adam had a tendency to use his face to stop the fists of his high school classmates with whom he had intellectual disagreements. If I remember correctly it had something to do with him being the smart aleck Jewish kid in a Catholic school for boys. Now 60, he was having trouble breathing and it was disturbing his sleep and keeping him from getting quality rest. The same method that I used to optimize for spine surgery worked to help Adam quickly and fully recover from surgery to fix his oft broken nose. Whether a broken back or a broken nose, seven of us were suffering and seven of us got better.

You already met our hiker, Doug Amend, who fell off a mountain. The little slice I gave you of his story was just the tip of a really scary iceberg, or more precisely glacier. The details of his story follow and underline how Doug's excellent physical conditioning was a lucky coincidence that more than likely saved his life and most certainly helped him to achieve a full recovery. Doug is a mortgage banker in Bend, Oregon. I interviewed him on the phone for a little over an hour. This is his story in his own words. If you are afraid of heights, brace yourself—it's a long way down.

> We were hiking. It was a fall day, 70 degrees, Sunday morning where myself and two co-workers had planned a few weeks before to do my annual Broken Top Summit after Labor Day. So, for the last four years in a row, I would hike up Broken Top to the Summit, free climbing. Roughly 8,700 feet is the area we would aspire to get to. Going in on the east side there is a lake that they call No Name Lake, and when we got to the edge of the lake at the base of the Summit, one of my co-workers and I navigated the scree field heading to the north, while the other co-worker decided, "Nope. Not gonna do it. You can't make me. I'm gonna walk around the lake; I'll meet you on the other side."

Doug adds with a laugh, "And we can identify him as the smart friend, absolutely."

> So, he hikes around the lake. We're in visual contact. We navigate the scree field. My not-so-smart co-worker slips on the snow that is on this northeast face, that doesn't get a lot of sun, and gets a little road rash on the back of his leg as he slides towards the lake. We get over to the ridge on the far side of the lake, meet up again, and I explained to both of them, "Okay. Here's where I want to go up to get to the peak." Smart partner looks and goes, "There's no way I'm going to do that." I explained to him, "Hey, I've done this three years in a row. Previously, I've gone up that path. This is a new path for me. I'm trying for a higher peak. This is my motivation." He looks up and says, "Good luck. I'm going to the lake. I'm going to go swimming. It's 32 degrees in the water."
>
> My not-so-smart friend, looks at me and he looks at him and he looks at me and he says "I'm going swimming," and off he goes. So, they traverse down the hill towards the lake and I start going up the ridge towards the summit. I got to a position where, free-climbing, I couldn't go any higher. I decided I wasn't going to go back down the way I came up. I'm going to go over on the other side, which was the north side. My feet got into some slurry, for lack of a better word. I mean it was really slushy, as my feet started to go out from underneath me. I'm looking around going, okay, well, this

isn't good. I'm trying to get back up. I can't gain any traction. I'm slowly sliding down, and at this point, I come to the conclusion, okay, I'm not going to be able to get back up here. It's relatively vertical at this point, at the top of the glacier. I was able to hold on to the edge of the ice to try to support myself, but, again, the weight without any traction, I couldn't pull myself up to gain any appreciable stability. And at that point, I rolled over onto my back, and with my right hand, I was hanging on to the gap, left hand was out in the air, feet were trying to dig into the glacier. I looked down at the rocks below and said to myself, so, this isn't good.

As I lost my grip my right foot hooked a small boulder. Sliding down the glacier headfirst, I quickly spun and got back to feet first. I knew that was the first thing I needed to do. As I was picking up speed, my heels were kicking up ice and dirt into my glasses so that I couldn't see. I was able to lift my glasses up, and, again, I am sliding at, you know, good speed. I don't know that I would call it break-neck speed, but it was, for all intents and purposes, it was about a 75-degree angle and I was sliding down from a vertical. I lift up my glasses; I see I'm going to go off the edge of the glacier. My next thought is pick your arms and legs up. You don't want to land on them because you'll break them, and, so, I went into helicopter mode. This I did consciously. I looked. I saw the edge. I knew I was going to go off into the air and I thought, yep, I don't want to do that. So, I lifted my

> arms and legs up, went off the edge and then dropped into that scree field onto my backpack, which had a pair of binoculars in it, and completely knocked all the wind out of me. Then I bounced out of that, got back up onto the glacier. It was basically a hole in the glacier and then rolled down to the rock pile that was mid-mountain and ended up face down in the fetal position.
>
> At that point, when I hit the scree field, that was the black for me, knocked the wind out of me. That was basically the last conscious thought. I don't really remember how I got into the fetal position. I just know from when I looked back up the mountain, when I regained my composure, I could see what I fell into and then how I got out of it and got to where I ended up. I'm thinking, okay, well, I can breathe. It hurts a fair amount, so I started wiggling my fingers on my left hand. Then I wiggled the fingers on my right hand. I felt my face and I'm like, huh, my head doesn't hurt; somehow, I didn't hit my head. I wasn't wearing a helmet. I extended my arms and I thought, okay, well, apparently I'm not paralyzed in the upper body. I wiggled my toes and started to flex my knees. I thought, wow, how did I do that? How did I fall that far and not break something? Then while trying to breathe, I go, nope, I broke my ribs.

How it is that Doug didn't die on impact is the first amazing part. Like I said in the previous chapter, what happens next with the search and rescue personnel is on the crazy side of stunning.

But, I guess "rules is rules" when you're delivering emergency services.

Doug very evenly continued,

> Then I called 911, because at that point, I'm like, yeah, I'm not going to be able to hike out. They took the information and switched me to Search and Rescue who basically says, "Hey, I can see where you are on the side of the hill, based on the ping. Where were you when you fell?" I said, "At the top." He goes, "Well, if you don't have a life-threatening injury, you can see, and you didn't break any arms or legs, we're not coming to get you."
>
> Doug countered saying, "I don't know that I need a med flight, but it would be nice if I could get somebody to come up here with a four-wheeler and get me out of here, because I don't think I can hike out." They just said, "Well, nope, we can't do it. Med flight or four-wheeler, you're on BLM [Bureau of Land Management] property, you have to have a life-threatening injury or be incapacitated. You're not. Do you have a first aid kit?" I said, "Yes, I do." He says, "Well, look in it for Ibuprofen. I'd take a couple of those to help with the rib pain and, you know, start hiking."

I just have to make another comment here. How do you tell a person who just fell 300 feet off a mountain to take an aspirin and start walking? Warning, it gets worse from here.

Doug takes a long pause, "Took me eight hours."

Some back injuries from trauma really don't manifest fully for a couple of days. I know that was my experience after the car accident that injured me. Now Doug's story turns toward the aftermath of the fall. It is important to follow Doug's journey of wanting to be okay, only to find out that he had a long and painful road ahead of him that would require the intervention of a spine surgeon.

Doug is matter-of-fact in the telling, but I could tell the recollection was painful.

> It was the T11 vertebrae in a burst fracture, so when I got in the emergency room, the doctor assessed me saying, "Well, there's nothing we really can do for broken ribs. Your arms are black and blue. You've got a nice road rash on your left butt cheek. We'll go ahead and order an X-ray as a precaution. Okay. Well, we got some bad news. You didn't break any ribs, but you broke your back."

In Chapter 4, "What Are My Options," Doug continues his story recounting the effort he made looking for information about the easiest path to getting better. Predictably, every one of the spine patients at our gathering tells the same story of the "good news, bad news" of doing research about their injury on the Internet. That's another part of what happened—nearly scaring ourselves away from surgery by searching the Internet. More about that later.

Doug suffered a trauma and knew immediately that he had really hurt himself. At the other end of the spectrum is our young violinist, Joy H. Sometimes back issues creep up on patients over a long period of time. Her pain was just as bad as Doug's, but it came about in a totally different way. Joy, as I mentioned, was candid and open about the fact that her pain was so severe that she actually considered suicide. Let me add something here about that solution. I was fortunate many years ago to work with the Suicide Prevention Hotline. Their standard line to dissuade callers from taking their lives is, "A permanent solution to a temporary problem is never a good idea."

This is how Joy tells her story:

> It began when I was 11 years old. I started playing the violin at that time. That is the reason we missed it. We missed all the signals. I knew I was having pain, but we associated it with the price that budding musicians pay. My back hurt, usually only when I practiced my violin, and it would go away after. Sometimes it would linger if I practiced more and more, as I grew into the profession. Sometimes it would still be there in the evening, and my mom would rub my back. I never really thought much about it; it just kinda crept up. It got gradually worse, until about the time I was 18. I had just finished high school, I was teaching the violin and playing and performing full-time. One day I had had a particularly long day, nine hours of teaching and playing. I got in my car to drive home, and the pain . . . I guess it just penetrated through my thoughts, and I realized, "I'm in chronic pain." I didn't notice. It kind of got me all of a sudden. I think as a kid, you just do what you've got to do to make it through, and I hadn't really stopped to consider what normal was like. I was really afraid. I had a hard time moving my arms to drive myself home.

> I was afraid I wouldn't be able to drive myself home. Sheer willpower got me through that car ride. I talked to my parents. I said, "Okay, we need to see somebody, this is really serious, and my friends who play the violin aren't going through this. I guess it's not normal." That was the start. Initially, my parents were on board, they said, "Yeah, let's go see somebody." So, we went to see a doctor. I believe the first one we saw was a shoulder specialist. We didn't know it was the back. We just assumed, because of the violin, it should be a shoulder issue. So, we went to see a shoulder specialist, and he took an X-ray, and he said, "Hey, by the way, do you know your back is bent?"

At this point I asked Joy if she had scoliosis.

> No, it was technically a deformity that wasn't classed as scoliosis, but we didn't find that out at the time. People were calling it scoliosis, but they didn't really know what to do with it. They just said, "This isn't bad enough for you to be in pain; you should just deal with it." I got a myriad of answers from the host of doctors that we saw after that first guy. They just said, "Yeah, it shouldn't be hurting you." But they did explain traditional scoliosis curvatures, and that if it's not past a certain curvature, it shouldn't be painful, and "people deal with this all the time." Finally, I just said, "That's why I'm here. I am in pain. This isn't going away, it's getting worse." It was a fight to be heard. I was the only one in my corner, honestly.

I couldn't be rationalized with . . . I can't even explain the thoughts in my head during that period. I was looking for surgery all along, honestly. I asked pretty much every doctor I talked to, "Can you please fix this, just operate." They had a variety of reasons for saying no. Most of them would say something like, "You're too young to have this surgery now." I think more what they were trying to say would be, "If you start having this type of fusion now it won't be good for you." Every time you have a fusion, there's the effect that you have an adjacent level failure, someday. That's really common knowledge. They would explain something like "If you have it now, in 5 to 10 years, you'll probably need an extension of that fusion. By the time you're really old, you'll have most of your back fused." I was going to start with T1 through T7. That's a significant amount of my thoracic spine. Expanding that on either side, every 10 years, it was going to look pretty gnarly by the end. I see what they were saying. It's only been four years since my operation, but so far I haven't had any adjacent level issues. I've tried to take really good care of my back, because I want to avoid more surgery if at all possible. It's probably likely, down the road. The thing is, I think it should've been my choice. I knew the risks of it. I thought, "Yep, it's probably going to need more surgeries, but how old do I have to get . . . how old and miserable do I have to be before you'll do this operation?" That was the question I finally asked: "I'm missing the

> prime of my life here, suffering away in pain. What's the magic number, what do you want me to be, before I have this?"

I think it is important to underline what we are hearing from Joy.

There may be a difference between the wisdom of a patient versus the concerns of a doctor.

Dr. Justin Saliman agrees that the patient sometimes knows what is best.

> There is something to be said for patient instinct, and I do think that the patients who do their research, get second opinions and listen to every opinion, and then choose the surgeon in this case who seems like is making the most sense, honestly – that's probably the most important thing. Which one, when they talk, makes the most sense, and you can kind of understand, and it seems like they're going to get you the best outcome, and you go with them. Be paranoid enough that you're doing research and getting multiple opinions. But don't be so paranoid that you never make a decision.

It is a crucial point when you think about the difference between how a doctor sees your problem and how you do. The doctor is almost certainly correct from a medical perspective on the facts, but *you* may be emotionally correct on what is right for you. More about that later too.

In the previous chapter we heard Robert G. talk about the toll those 30 years of walking on concrete at his place of business took on his back. You may recall that a sneeze set off a series of events that ultimately resulted in Robert needing back surgery. Something he said during the interview struck me as ironic and oddly familiar. See if you catch it in his statement, "At the time I was quite physically fit. I was in martial arts and so exercising daily, stretching daily. I was in probably one of the best times of fitness in my life. And, it literally started all from that. I mean, obviously something was going on because I don't think just a sneeze would cause that to happen."

Yes, he was quite physically fit. Wait a second—so was our hiker, Doug Amend. I was bicycling 40 miles around Los Angeles every weekend before I got hurt. In fact, we were all in excellent physical condition, and yet we all suffered crippling back pain. What happened? A trauma, a deformity, a degenerative disc disease were all part of what happened to each of us. It is likely that you could tell your own story and it would include some or all of these factors. The reason I am emphasizing the fact that we were all fairly physically fit is because it seems to be a key component to optimizing for surgery. Being physically fit means different things for different people. I want you to focus on that aspect of these patients' experiences because our doctors and physical therapists have some very strong opinions about how crucial physical readiness is to optimizing for surgery.

After her second child, Linda B. started to have back pain out of the blue. Linda remembers how surprised she was when her doctor said:

> "Wow, you have severe degenerative disc disease, which is unusual for your age." At that time I think I

> was 37. And he said, "You would benefit from a spinal fusion."

That's another important fact that is important to note. Linda's back problems, like our young violinist, Joy, were unusual for patients at their age. If you are thinking that you are too young for issues with your back and what happened to them can't happen to you, it might be in your best interest to reconsider. Sometimes, what happens in your back happens slowly and silently over a long period of time until a sneeze or a pregnancy brings it to the surface.

Lucio D., like Doug Amend and me, suffered a high impact trauma. Lucio was hit so hard from behind in his car accident that it actually tore his stomach lining. Lucio reported,

> The first set of surgeries, 'cause I had several injuries, the first set of surgeries happened in 2016. It was a minor surgery, a laparoscopic surgery of my abdomen, the fascia between my stomach and my hip tore open and my stomach wanted to come out. I was hit that hard. That surgery had to be done immediately because I could barely walk around or do anything. So, I went from being extremely healthy, you know, a guy who could grab a surfboard and go surfing for hours, to barely being able to go to the bathroom. That's how awful it was.

Again, notice that Lucio was in good physical condition before he got hurt. His body was in optimal shape and he was an "optimized" patient without even knowing what that meant. Lucio and I discussed how fortunate it was that he was eating well and was active before the accident. The same was true of Doug Amend. In fact, all of the patients, except for me, were very careful about their diet before they even knew they should be. I found out about the key role of nutrition years into struggling with healing and getting my energy back. It made an extraordinary difference in the latter part of my recovery and it will for you too. More about that in Chapter 11, "Fire Up The Recovery Engine!"

So, what happened? Six patients, a hiker, a mother, a violinist, an entrepreneur, a retiree and a writer all made a date with a surgeon for six different reasons. They all had reservations about seeing the spine doctor. They all struggled for months and, in some cases, for years with chronic pain until the surgeons intervened. And they all got well and recovered in a variety of ways. What we learned from their collective experience is that there were common threads for what makes a good patient. Those common threads were validated not just by the patients, but by the surgeons, physical therapists, chiropractor, and nutritionist. I have simply put a name to our collective experience as a path for getting well. Simply put, we were all accidentally optimized patients.

These stories, the experiences of actual spine surgery patients, are detailed here to help you gain some context about what happened to you, either over time from disease or deformity or from sudden trauma. Over 600,000 patients each year face the challenge before you–to commit to getting better and overcoming their limitations and chronic pain, or to decide to just to live with them. What happened to each of us should give you some insight into what is happening to you and what your options are. What you learn here won't make the physical and mental challenges of spine surgery any less painful. But, I am fairly confident that we may be able to help relieve some of your anxiety, help you to develop a confident and positive mental attitude, give you the tools you need to determine what is best for you, and provide some action items to help your body heal as quickly and fully as possible.

If those of us who are contributing to this book do our job well, you will know whether or not spine surgery - or any surgery - is right for you. There is something instructive in hearing the journey of others. There is also something comforting and reassuring about realizing, "Hey, that's what happened to me too!" More important is knowing that the patients whose stories you are hearing all survived and recovered fully from their disease or injury. So much of what I learned writing this book grew out of me asking, "What happened to you?" But, that question went beyond hearing about a fall off a mountain, a sneeze that finally brought a big man down, or pregnancy with a second child that left mom with a damaged back. But, "what happened" also extended to how to find a doctor, what worked in rehab, how long it took to recover, what the challenges were in the hospital and at home right after surgery and then in rehab. All of that is what's on the table when patients gather to talk about what happened.

In the most elementary way, what happened to me is that I was injured. One way or another, that's what happened to you too. I tried everything in the world to stop the pain. I found out the same thing happened to the other five spine patients sitting at the table. I finally gave in and realized it was time to see the spine doctor. Yup, same thing happened to them. In a little bit of a different way, the same thing happened with Adam when he bit the bullet and decided to fix a decades old problem with is nose. When I got home I realized there were going to be a number of serious challenges relating to bending, twisting and lifting, affectionately known by the acronym BLT. We all struggled with dressing, bathing, and preparing food because of that. Every patient recovering from any major injury of any sort has some kind of functional challenge. Those challenges can have serious mental consequences as well that are not as obvious as the cast, or crutch or sling.

And the most difficult experience we shared was learning all of this the hard way—after we needed to know it.

After reading this book, the experience of being unprepared won't be an experience you will have shared with us. What happened? We were all needlessly unprepared for surgery because we weren't lucky enough to have a room full of people to walk us through the blow by blow of what happened to them. Chances are very high what happened to us is going to happen to you—including a full recovery.

In the next chapter you will learn no one really wants to go see the surgeon. We all searched for an alternative, any alternative, to what is rumored to be the "horror" of spine surgery, if we're to believe what we read on the Internet. At some point in every one of our stories, there came a moment when the daily over-the-counter painkiller, physical therapy, chiropractic, and everything else you can image just wasn't going to do the job anymore. Our team will tell us about what the alternatives are and how to know if surgery is going to work for you—or not. One of the physical therapists talks about a highly effective aqua therapy, which will either relieve your back pain or confirm to you that it's time to see the surgeon. We are excited about sharing what we have learned and encourage you to get a pen or pencil and make notes in the margins!

4

WHAT ARE MY OPTIONS?

This might be your favorite chapter if you are hoping to avoid surgery. The conversation is moving on from talking about what happened to what we did about it. Like the many different causes of back pain, we all tried many different options before we made the trip to see the surgeon. You may be luckier than any one of us and not need surgery at all. But, how do you know if you do or if you don't? There are many options from aqua therapy to chiropractic to epidurals. This is the twilight zone for back pain that most people know little or nothing about. If you are researching alternatives to surgery on the Internet, be warned. Much of what you will find on Google is 5% information and 95% marketing. The patients and doctors who are sharing their experiences in this book have a lot to say about whether or not they found realistic and viable options in lieu of surgery. The good news about their comments and information: no marketing. They have nothing to sell. The only things they have to offer are insights and options. The Optimized Patient is focused on patient education to give you the knowledge you need to manage your best outcome.

Please don't confuse what you would prefer not to do with what you really need to do. I think our mom, Linda B., very concisely summed up the patient's desire of wanting to avoid spine surgery. She had already gotten a doctor's opinion that she needed and would achieve pain relief with back surgery. Like so many people suffering from back pain, one opinion was exactly that, one opinion. Remember what Linda said?

> Real bad back pain, and it was often. And I don't recall if the leg pain started then? I think it did. Yeah, because that's one of the indicators of whether they can help you or not, and of how severe you are. So, I got the second opinion; they said the same thing. And at that time I had a brand-new baby and a toddler. And it was the first time I had heard the word "back surgery." But most of what I remember is the back pain.
>
> I did every single modality in the book. Well not every single one, but I tried quite a few. Chiropractic helped me along the way. Oh, and I remember I got my first steroid shot; it was such a simple thing. He said, "Oh, I can give you a steroid shot," and I lifted up my shirt, bent over, and he gave me an easy shot in the back. That helped for years. That got me through quite a few years. Along with chiropractic, stretching, exercise . . . what else did I do? Ibuprofen, not all the time, though, because if you keep using that it doesn't work anymore either.

As you will hear from the other patients, that is the journey.

We all tried anything, everything, before either seeing or saying "yes" to the surgeon.

That certainly was my journey. My first stop was the chiropractor. After all, I got slammed around in a car crash and common sense dictated that my back was out of alignment. And it was out of alignment. But, that was only a small part of the story. At one of my adjustments the chiropractor asked me to stand up on my toes. At that moment and I am talking about months after the car accident, I realized that I was seriously hurt. Sure, I was limping from the pain, but it never occurred to me to try to stand up on my toes. I had lost complete muscle control in my calves! Did I rush off to see the spine surgeon? Heck no! I went to the pain management specialist for epidurals. One was supposed to do the job. After the second epidural I was still at 8 on the pain scale. After four epidurals, the pain did stop. My limp continued, but the pain did stop—though I still couldn't get up on my toes. But, ok, at least the pain had stopped and I was healing.

Oddly, it was a urinary tract infection that ultimately put me in front of a spine surgeon. As odd as that may sound to you as a patient, it makes total sense to spine doctors. It's called drop foot. The same nerves that drive your calves also drive your bladder. So, when my urologist noted on a sonogram that my bladder was not emptying properly he knew it was a back problem. The medical term is a neurogenic bladder. Now, with this new knowledge, spine surgery was no longer an option—it was a life-saving medical necessity. Once I picked the doctor and set a date, the optimization of this patient began.

Even though Doug Amend fell off a mountain, he was not interested in rushing off to the surgeon's office. Doug tells it this way:

> So they do the CT scan, and they said, "No internal injuries but you didn't just break your back you got a burst fracture and there's shrapnel around your spinal cord. We're going to have to do surgery." At that point, I asked who was on call. They said, "Dr. Hadden." I said, "You tell Tony to put me in a back brace; I'll go see him later this week." (It happened that Doug had a professional and personal relationship with the doctor on call.) "I don't think we're going to do surgery tonight." The doctor says, "They'll never let you out of the hospital."

But they called Dr. Hadden who, knowing Doug well, said, "No, if that's what he wants, put him in a brace and send him home."

Predictably, Doug was immediately crystal clear that he did not want to rush into surgery. The back brace was "Plan A," surgery was "Plan B." Doug and I laughed about hoping for the best. We both skipped over preparing for the worst. Doug continued,

> I was in a back brace for six weeks until the next appointment. I was doing a lot of research. There was a study done that patients had similar results using only a back brace versus going in and doing surgery. Dr. Hadden confirmed that he didn't think that it was an effective treatment even though there was a medical research paper on it. I said, "Hey, why not," so he tried it on me. And here we sit six weeks later going okay, that didn't

> work. We're going to have to go in and do the surgery anyway.

You know the saying, "100% you will miss the shot you never take." Doug took a shot, we all took our shot. Sometimes taking a shot does work. There is a ray of light. Solomon Joseph, a physical therapist at Advanced Orthopedic and Sport Physical Therapy leads a three-times-a-week aqua therapy class in Long Beach, California. Of all the surgical avoidance strategies I have heard about over seven years, his is the most sensible and most effective. Solomon shared his view about how to use a swimming pool to either relieve your pain or optimize you for surgery. Solomon advised,

> For prehab, if they're trying to avoid surgery, they should just get into the water to build up endurance and strength. Of course, they work on strengthening because they're not trying to ruin the surgery, so to speak. So, they can get in there and have pain be their guide, as far as moving and jumping around and exercising and building strength while they're unloaded in the water system. Usually when they get in the water, a lot of the pain dissipates and they can actually do more. They can strengthen the muscles more. The water will give resistance; the faster they try to move in the water, the more resistance it will give them. And they can use tools like paddles and boards, kick boards, to increase resistance and build strength and endurance to try to help stabilize the muscles around the spine to prevent surgery.

I had to stop Solomon there. Even though I was in his classes for rehab, I had no idea that his methodology was also excellent for either relieving back pain so you don't need surgery or optimizing your core for surgery if the pain does not subside. To make sure I was hearing him correctly I asked, "So what you're saying is, there's no downside, that it in no way compromises a good outcome in surgery. There's no bad outcome from getting in the pool prior to surgery?"

Solomon went a little deeper for clarification:

> That's right. If they're trying to avoid surgery, it's just you get into the water to build up endurance and strength. If it's like major bulges from the disks, there's not a whole lot anybody can do for that without surgery. This is where we get into the prehab before surgery, to build up strength and conditioning to get ready for surgery because it takes a lot of pressure off the spine, off the bulge and everything else, so the muscles can work and build up strength. Because people really can't do a whole lot outside, they get weaker if they're not exercising and moving around. Getting in the water promotes strength, endurance, and core stabilization prior to surgery. And it helps with the rehab after surgery.

That is a remarkable revelation that I have shared with many people who are considering back surgery. I wish I had known this before my surgery. It is a key and hopeful note for anyone who is hoping to recover from any kind of injury without surgery.

In simplest terms, either one of two things is going to happen: You're either going to condition up and perhaps avoid surgery, or condition up and be better prepared to go through the surgery.

Robert G. wouldn't consider spine surgery until he was ready to retire from his automobile service business. On one hand we get that, but 20 years is a long time to work through your options. Robert remembers it this way,

> And thinking 20 years ago, I'm just summarizing this, that if I had disc disease then I would have had a lot more problems, been out more frequently since that time.

Robert had a strategy and it did not include spine surgery. Robert said,

> Yeah, numerous times I've taken cortisone shots. Throughout that time period I had three different times where I had cortisone shots. And, there were epidurals, two or three times in thinking back. To be honest, I couldn't tell you if it was just the cortisone shot at first or the epidural later. I don't remember how the sequence went with it. But, once I'd first gotten that shot I felt like a new man."

That was the beginning of Robert's journey. I asked him to give me some perspective on the time frame, how old he was when the pain began? He said, "About 35 years old. Yeah, that was the onset of the pain and suffering for years to come. Twenty years before I decided to finally have it done, yes. Or 18 years, I guess, 18 years." I asked him if he tried anything other than the cortisone shots. Robert recalled, "I did. I went to chiropractors. Later, actually during that, I would say about a nine-month period, when that first shot really helped me out; I again, was very active. And the pain was gone so I could just forget about it, you know. I mean, it just went away—I literally had no pain. Still doing martial arts and still active, but I did go to a chiropractor infrequently. And I wouldn't say necessarily for the lower back pain that I was having at that time, but just from pain in the back and shoulders, more from sparring and different things I was doing."

> I just got out of bed one morning and the same thing happened to me. I got up incorrectly, I guess, and locked my back up again. This time I was down for probably about four days. Went back in and did more testing and they had suggested then to have surgery, but I just wasn't confident in technology, I think, was a big part of it. And, the other part is, I had four boys I was raising and I was active in work and in the prime of my career. I just didn't feel that I was ready to have that done. So, then I have another injection and I'm fine, literally. Once I had the injections, it felt like it cured me. I would say another couple of months later, two to three months later, I started to have consistent pain, but not to where it locked up and I couldn't move, but just to the point where it felt like somebody was jabbing me in my lower back. I would say a couple of months after the second injection. And, it was chronic day and night where I was not sleeping well. I'm not one for taking pills and drugs. So, to be honest with you, I just lived through it through all the years until ultimately the third time it came about, and then I had another injection. I want to say that was probably about two years before my surgery, which I ended up having, and that lasted about a day

> and a half, to where I had no pain. And, then it all came back with a vengeance—more acute pain or chronic pain consistently day and night no matter what I did. I really wanted to hold off until I was going to retire—March of this year—but it just got to the point where when I did go to work (and in my work I'm literally on my feet 10 to 12 hours every day), I couldn't stand for more than five minutes.

At the other end of the spectrum is our young violinist, Joy H. Even though she ultimately challenged the doctors about delaying surgery, she also ran the gamut of exhausting her options. Joy recalls,

> I tried a lot of things. I had multiple stints of physical therapy. It felt like every new doctor wanted to prescribe a new physical therapy routine, so I did a lot of physical therapy. Almost every time they discharged me early, they were just like "We're not helping you. This is torture for us as much as it is for you." So, they would discharge me. We tried medications, eventually. I got married in the middle of all this, and the pain kept escalating. I thought, "This isn't who I am, it's not me anymore. There is no hope to live like this." I was ready to take my life. Tim, my husband, said "Well, how about we try a pain specialist?" I researched a lot of specialists, honestly. Because I felt like we were still missing something big. But every time I would try a new medication, I would research things, natural things that should be doing what the chemical substance was doing. If it was

treating inflammation, I would research inflammation, how to control that naturally, just things to try."

Ultimately Joy did see the spine surgeon.

The doctors want to chime in at this point. They want you to make sure that the problem you have really is a spine problem and not just ordinary back trouble that actually does respond to non-surgical options. I asked Dr. Christopher Hills whose practice is in Jackson, Wyoming, if he recommended non-surgical strategies before committing to a surgical fix. Dr. Hills had many suggestions that may or may not work for you. Any and all of what he says should be discussed with your doctor who has specific knowledge of your situation. Dr. Hills offered,

> Well, the patient should have already been working with a physical therapist pre-surgery, and that most times should be transitioned into a home exercise regimen where the patient has had a very regular routine that they've worked on for their pre-hab, with core strengthening, aerobic conditioning, obviously the appropriate stretching and nerve block techniques, and then, again, it depends . . . I don't make every person do this, but I think if you want to work with an acupuncturist, dry needling, things of that nature. Pilates is a great one for patients to work in for core strength. Obviously, yoga has some benefits in it. You have to be able to modify many of the extreme positions in yoga to be able to accommodate for spine conditions, but it's just very critical that patients are actively engaged in strengthening their body."

I lead with Dr. Hill because it is important to note, as we learned earlier in this chapter from physical therapist Solomon Joseph, that sometimes the preparation becomes the cure.

That sentiment is echoed by Dr. Sanjay Khurana who was my surgeon in Marina del Rey, California. I had discussed with Dr. Khurana that I had worked with a chiropractor and previously had four epidurals from a pain specialist. None of that had done any good. I asked him to comment on my case. I think what he said may be instructive for you. Dr. Khurana pointed out,

> So, my mission was to find the appropriate solution, whether it be non-surgery or surgery. The clarification for me, in terms of whether or not you had much delay of any conservative modalities was pretty clear. I did not think non-surgery had any role in you. Because at your age, which was pretty young (61 at that time), and with your expectations of quality of life, I did think there was a huge upside to simply removing the stenosis that you had at both those levels.

This brings me back to my suggestion that you should review your other options with a surgeon. I might have spared myself a lot of needless pain and expense by accepting the surgical fix sooner than later.

The chiropractor would seem to be the first port of call for most people suffering from back pain. But, how do you know what kind of chiropractor to see? How do you even know what questions to ask to get moving in the right direction? It is important to note here that unlike physical therapy and surgery, your insurance may not cover treatment from a chiropractor. I personally had a disappointing experience with chiropractic for two reasons. Ten treatments, although expertly delivered, did not relieve my symptoms. Even though the chiropractor worked in concert with my spine surgeon to avoid a third surgery, the efforts to fix a bulging disc did not self-correct. A third surgery was ultimately required. I endured two months of pain in the optimistic hope that my back would heal on its own, but it did not. Secondarily, that opened up a year-long skirmish with my insurance carrier to try to get the chiropractor paid. That said, you may get relief and be able to avoid surgery. If you want to try to travel this road, here are some things I learned from my practitioner to help you get the best possible result.

You should meet a few practitioners before you make a choice. There are a variety of ways they treat. You can ask, "What is the premise of your practice?" The world of chiropractic is broken down into two approaches. One is known as "straight" and the other is known as "mixer." A straight chiropractor will look at the biomechanics of a spinal failure, determine what are the factors causing the problem and then treat specifically for that problem. The mixers may also utilize colonics, crystals, and the sorts of things we associate with Eastern medicine. The mixer is a little more ethereal and holistic, rather than addressing the biomechanical issue of a single joint with a specific problem and all the mechanics around that joint and disc segment.

Straight chiropractors also practice in two different ways, either employing general manipulation or specific manipulation. In my case, the chiropractor was a specific practitioner who looked at the joints up and down, above and below where the damaged disc was.

The goal is to figure out what happened to the biomechanics of that area and how to specifically restore symmetry and alignment and open up the disc space and give the joint room to breathe. From my discussions I learned that it is always a good thing to increase range of motion before and after surgery.

The chiropractor should be able to tell you what went wrong biomechanically from looking at an MRI and an X-ray. The practitioner should offer his opinion on how to help it and how long it may take to get it to stabilize and return to proper alignment. The chiropractor should also offer how many treatments it may take to maintain a healthy disc. But, what if it doesn't work as planned—as happened with me? After everything has been tried to avoid surgery, how do you make the decision to see a surgeon?

We all know that there's a problem with doing the same thing over and over again and expecting a different outcome. Your suffering is not going to end if you keep doing the same thing. Thinking it will change is simply insane. I allowed six weeks to give the disc a chance to breathe and heal. I knew at the last treatment that surgical intervention was needed to stop the pain. Twenty-four hours after an outpatient discectomy I was pain free and on the road to a full recovery. Does chiropractic help? Best answer, it couldn't hurt, except for the bill.

If you are reading this book you are more than likely researching the Internet directly to learn what the options might be in the first place. Dr. Google is another source of information. By that I mean, going to the Internet to learn what can be done. Remembering that we are sitting at a table with all of the patients, if you had eyes on them you would see them all smirking and shaking their heads at the mention of the Internet. Personally, I asked my nephew, who is an anesthesiologist, what he would recommend. That is how I found my way to a pain management specialist. I did, however, spend significant time on the Internet trying to understand what might help in combination with chiropractic and other options. All my research did was frighten me . . . as it did all the other patients. This is a key piece of insight that should help you to make better decisions about how to navigate the voyage to fully being you again.

Our mountain climber, Doug Amend, did his homework with the help of his spine surgeon. His recollection actually made me laugh.

> I'm on my tablet looking. Okay, they tell me I broke my T11; how can I fix it? Then I'm going down the rabbit hole of here's burst fracture treatments and then here's some studies and then you just keep going down that hole finding information, you know, because **I'm on the Internet scaring the crap out of myself** and he sent me the link, and I said, "Yep, that did it. That scared me." If that's the surgery that I'm trying to avoid, how can I do it?

Linda B., whose back pain began after her second child also found her way to the Internet and found no comfort there. Linda had an interesting insight as to why the Internet may be distressing. Linda said,

> I went to two different orthopedics, and one neurologist. So, I had five experts over the course of eight years tell me that I would benefit from this surgery. And

> I learned that I needed to stay away from the Internet. I learned that there was a lot of negative information, as far as people went. For me, that meant if you're happy, you're not usually making notes and comments on the Internet, but if you're in pain you have time to complain, and just not complain, but express your distress.

We all know that people are more likely to post about a disappointment than they are about a success. That is unfortunate, but it is human nature.

I want to encourage anyone reading this book to thoroughly explore all of your options. As we have learned, there are a lot of them. In hindsight, if I had known at the beginning of my journey what I know now, I would have passed on all the non-surgical options. Once I understood and accepted that surgery was not just another option, but was essential, the idea to optimize was born. The four rounds of epidurals did not fix the problem. Months with the chiropractor did not fix the problem. Yes, I got temporary relief and the joy of believing that I had dodged the surgical bullet. But, in the end all that I did was delaying the needed correction in the architecture of my back so my body, could do what it is programmed to do: heal. Stopping the pain is not fixing the problem. Clearly, that was the experience of Robert G. and Linda B. and Joy H. as well. We all got the shots, and the adjustments, and took the pills we needed to kill the pain, but it took the skilled work of the surgeon to create the opportunity to heal.

The strategy of walking in chest-high water suggested by physical therapist Solomon Joseph, will either relieve your back pain or better prepare you for surgery. More about that later. As any chiropractor will suggest, getting your back into alignment as best you can may not only relieve your pain, but may also help the spine surgeons to do their best work. Both of those activities contribute to the core of what this book is about, how to be an optimized patient. Physical Therapist Patti Sogaard, sums it up this way:

> If you've exhausted all treatment and it's no longer helping and the patient can no longer do their daily life, their functions in life, then they need to see a doctor and move on to some other type of medical care.

Now that you know about the options, I believe you will find clarity in the collective thought process of our patients, doctors and physical therapists as we talk about considering surgical intervention. Truly, it's a very big decision and not to be taken lightly. If you are anything like us, over the years you have heard many reports of disastrous spine surgeries. I was blunt in asking each of the three spine surgeons why those stories are so pervasive in news reports and on the Internet. They have a lot to say about that as we consider denial and fear and accepting a surgical fix.

5

FEAR AND DENIAL

Each and every one of the patients who gathered at the table all feared "the horror stories about surgery." This book would not be complete if I did not directly question the surgeons who have joined us and ask them to address the horror stories. There are a lot of options as alternatives to surgery, as we have just learned, and anyone facing surgery would be crazy not to try to find a way to get well without going under the knife. Sadly, the negative forces driving that search for an alternative to surgery are denial and fear. Denial is the harder of the two mindsets to address.

The original title of this chapter was "Accepting the Surgical Fix". I was very focused on the fact that the group of spine patients that I interviewed had done and tried anything and everything possible to avoid surgery. The question is, does any of that apply to injury recovery when there is no decision to be made about what to do. The accident essentially made the decision for you in the emergency room. Now all you have is the fear of whether or not you will recover. If you take away one single idea for reading this book it should be that what is going on in you head will determine whether or not you will have the recovery you are hoping for in your body.

How many people reading this book think they can achieve a full and speedy recovery without any help? "It's no big deal I am fine. Why is everyone making a Federal case of out of it?" Sadly, many people in recovery will deny how badly they are hurt and refuse the guidance and the physical therapy they need for a full recovery. Many times those patients become chronically ill because they never allow themselves the time and help they need to fully heal. The optimized patient concept looks at both sides of the recovery coin. On one side there are those people who think they can tough it out and go it alone. One the other side of that coin are those patients who want to get better, they just do know how or know who to ask or where to find the appropriate help.

So, whether you have had an accident, are preparing for or recovering from surgery, we all come to this experience with a mindset about how to recover. The fear of the unknown, of being in a completely new experience, unwilling to make frightening decisions or commit to hard actions because we are in denial often present the biggest obstacle to getting well.

All of us wanted to believe that our accident, our fall, our degenerative disc disease, our stenosis . . . could be fixed somehow without surgery.

We now know that in some cases it can be. If what we just heard about aqua-therapy might work for you, a swimming pool sure would be a lot more fun than surgery! Even after the options have been tried and pain persists, the fear factor remains and many patients with chronic back pain remain reluctant to consider accepting the surgical fix.

I can remember, from the time I was a child, hearing stories of surgical disasters in the news. Sometimes it was a story about the wrong leg or arm being amputated. Often it was a story about how spine surgery, meant to relieve chronic pain, resulted in the patient spending the rest of their life in a wheelchair! I believe we have all been affected by some version or combination of those stories over our lifetime even though these stories had nothing to do with any condition we had at the time. Now, with the availability of information and misinformation on the Internet, there is a spotlight on disastrous surgical outcomes without any clear understanding of why the patient who is reporting their disappointment—or outrage—had such a bad result. The assumption, and what we usually hear reported on the news, is that the medical team of doctors and nurses simply messed it up. I believe those horror stories are running in the back of the minds of every patient confronted with the need for spine surgery. The doctors told me that the fears expressed by patients are normal based on what the patients have heard or read. But, they say, the facts around why those stories exist need to be known to determine if they, in any way, relate to you, your condition, or the doctor whom you have chosen to fix your problem.

Perhaps, the perfect story to begin with was shared by our entrepreneur and star-gazer, Lucio D. Lucio, you may recall, was rear-ended in car accident while sitting at a traffic light. His path to the surgical fix begins when he regains consciousness at the scene of the accident. Lucio remembers,

> When I came to, there was a lot of pain immediately. I couldn't feel my legs. I felt like my back was broken. I couldn't move my left arm; it had totally gone numb. I didn't have broken bones or anything. But, then I realized that evening, they said, "We'd like to have you stay tonight." And I said, "No, I feel okay." And I walked away, I signed myself out. I was in the hospital for about ten hours. I said, "I'll be fine. I'll just walk away from this."

I would say that is a very clear case of denial. Once reality set in, denial was no longer an option and Lucio began to fear what was coming next. Lucio recalled:

> I went back to my home, I got in bed, just to lie down, and it was pretty late. And the next morning around 7, 8 o'clock, I'm calling to my daughter and a friend that I had over, I said, "Please, I can't even get out of this bed." I couldn't even move. And then it began: the slew of drugs that I had to take just to get myself moving. The doctor at the ER, who had the X-ray and MRIs done immediately, he came back to me with the report and he showed me an MRI scan and said, "You're going to need surgery on your neck. You're going to possibly need surgery on your lower back. You're definitely going to need surgery on that abdomen." And he's like, "I can let you walk away, this is not dire. You're not going to die here. But you're definitely going to have a hard time this next week. Please, go see your doctor immediately and get these surgeries." And I said, "Okay, I'll talk to

> my doctor." I just wanted to get out of the hospital. No one likes to stay in the emergency room hospital or intensive care unit for that long.

I asked Lucio if he did anything for pain management, did he get any painkillers. Remember, he is a very independent "get it done" sort of fellow. He quickly came back,

> Yeah, yeah, I already had some from a dental surgery I had some time before, and I said, "I'll just take some of these and I won't need a prescription." I saw my doctor immediately and he took a look at me, and he goes, "Yeah, you need some pain management." So, he started me on the pain management, and it was controlled a lot better. Well, we just stayed with muscle relaxers, and then we went to a painkiller that had acetaminophen and hydrocodone in it. And I don't like taking those because they make me feel out of it, so I would only take those if it was unbearable pain. Most of the time, I stayed on some muscle relaxers which were toward the evening. But I found that if I stayed still, it hurt even more and the numbness came on more. If I moved, it seemed to be a little bit better, but if I sat down, if I laid down, those days afterwards, it was awful. I couldn't get up. And the numbness was really scaring me. The left side of my body was totally, completely going numb at times. And I'm talking, like, half of my head. If you were to split me straight down, half my body was completely numb, like it had ants–you know, the tingly feeling like you have."

> Half my body would get that, and it was scary because my left eyeball and left ear and left ass cheek and my left foot would go numb. "Okay, this is not good." And then the pain got worse. Much, much worse. To the point where there were days where I was on my knees, head down between my knees, trying to stretch my back without feeling in some of the other extremities. Daily it was like a full-time job for me just to exist. And that's when I said, "Okay, this has to be done quick." But then with everything that fell along, you know, when you start telling your doctor, "Okay, I need this now, please. Get me to a surgeon." It doesn't happen overnight. When you hear that you're going to need surgery, the first thing you say to yourself is, "No, no, no. I don't want to be cut into and please let's look for an alternative." So, we went down that road at first, and I asked the surgeon and my doctor, I kept telling them, "Hey, please, before we go to surgery, let's please figure out a way that I don't have to do this."

Lucio's experience has within it all of our experiences on the way to accepting the surgical fix. Enduring pain that destroys your quality of life, hoping to relieve the pain with drugs and the body's own natural program to heal, realizing that is not going to happen, considering surgery and learning about all the horror stories, finally seeing a doctor and getting the reassuring information to commit to the surgical fix. That was exactly what happened to me. It wasn't until everything else had failed that I was lucky enough to have lunch with an attorney friend of mine who had just had the exact surgery I was considering. I have mentioned a couple of times in this book that my happy outcome sometimes had the element of dumb luck to it. Something as important as your spine surgery should not be reliant on dumb luck. That's why I am writing this book; to help you skip over all the mistakes all of us made and get you on the road to being optimized.

So, why are there so many horror stories? Who better to ask than the surgeons themselves? You can imagine that I had this very discussion with my surgeon quite directly. I asked Dr. Khurana to go on the record about why there is so much horrible lore around spine surgery. Without flinching he went right after it:

> There's a lot of technological innovation in imaging, a lot of progressive clinical studies that have demonstrated outcomes that we've kind of aggregated to come up with better solutions in understanding why certain interventions make patients worse, why certain interventions make patients better, and like you just touched on, a lot of times a clinical imaging success, like a perfect X-ray could have no correlation to the patient's clinical outcome. I think there are a lot of things that come into the mix from an input standpoint, like I mentioned originally. It has to do with the appropriate imaging, the correlation of imaging to symptoms, learning lessons from the history of nightmare surgeries. I think in the 70s, 80s, 90s, there's kind of a linear correlation with the magnitude of soft tissue stripping, kind of the invasiveness of surgery and actually the muscle trauma that comes with that, that we've identified as being bad

things for patient outcomes, that several innovative companies like Nuvasive[1] have essentially solved.

Kind of learning to strip the muscle of the spine less. A lot of Eugene Carragee's work, one of my mentors at Stanford, was identifying appropriate psychological profiles of patients that either correlate to bad or good outcomes. **Sometimes a patient's mindset could be so overwhelmed with depression or anxiety that no matter what the surgical pathology, you could almost predict a poor outcome.**

So, I think the correlation of knowing the physical issues of the spine, correlating that with a psychological profile of the patient, coupling that with technologically advanced ways to fix someone's body through less invasive means, it has really led to outcome profiles that are generally pretty good. Even if I look at taking an honest look at all my patients in the last 15 years, overall I can honestly say I've been very gratified with the overwhelming positive outcome of patients to surgery. Now, are there patients where it didn't quite pan out to where we wanted it to, and sometimes you can have unintended effects and complications, that is absolutely part of what we do, and it's part of any surgical field. But, when you look at your consecutive patient series about the recommendation for intervention and their outcomes, I think

---

1. www.nuvasive.com. Nuvasive is a manufacturer of medical devices. The hardware used in my fusions and the minimally invasive procedure used during my surgery were developed by Nuvasive. That is why his answer includes reference to that specific medical device company.

> overwhelmingly what I've done in my career, I think I've helped people 90, 95 percent plus of my patients, which has been very gratifying. It's been a great thing to see and I think we're standing on the shoulders of people who have learned lessons the hard way: perhaps by being well intended, but not doing the correct surgery, perhaps by doing the wrong surgery, perhaps by doing a surgery which is too invasive, perhaps by using imaging too heavily and not correlating to the patient's symptoms. But there are a lot of lessons that we've all collectively learned as spine surgeons to try to do the best for our patients. And it's additive. It requires a lot of things that have led to this kind of funneling of patient selection coupled with the appropriate surgical intervention, which has changed dramatically, even since the time I was training. I was training from the late 90s up until 2002. Even the way that I see things done now has very little correlation to the way it was done when I was in training. It has changed significantly.

It is important to underline that Dr. Khurana mentions patient psychology as part of the equation. If *The Optimized Patient* is about anything, it's about making sure you **go confidently and well prepared into your surgery**. There is no place for fear and denial in the equation of working confidently on your recovery. If we are hearing Dr. Khurana, that really could be the difference between a successful surgery and another horror story. As the conversation continues you will increasingly hear about your role in obtaining a successful outcome. The first step is making the decision to allow a surgeon to assess your situation for surgery. Once the surgery is done, the real work begins.

Dr. Justin Saliman echoed the importance of patient psychology,

> The funny thing is mental health relates to every subspecialty, as well. So, if you're talking about orthopedics, no matter what the subspecialty of orthopedics, be it spine or joint replacements or orthopedic sports or foot, ankle or hand or pediatrics or anything, really. There are even studies that have shown in shoulder surgery that depression has more to do with the outcome than in terms of if you take a depression assessment, the correlation between patients who are depressed and getting better, there's a direct relationship. So, if a patient is depressed, then they are less likely to get better from rotator cuff repair surgery than patients who are not depressed.[2]

Think about how stunning that statement is. I have to confess that when Dr. Saliman first told me about this study I couldn't imagine it was as strong he was presenting it. I have footnoted the link so you can find it and read it for yourself. If fear, denial and depression are driving your choices, the research says you may be diminishing your chances of a full recovery.

Dr. Vermon Esplin is a senior hand surgeon in Eastern Idaho. After 31 years in practice he notes some patterns in good or bad patient outcomes.

---

2. https://www.researchgate.net/publication/343352090_Effect_of_anxiety_and_depression_on_early_pain_and_range_of_motion_after_rotator_cuff_repair_-_measured_by_HADS_Hospital_Anxiety_and_Depression_Scale_-

> I think it goes back to the motivation is the key. Some people also in life have had things done for them. They have really not had too many challenges to overcome, and all of a sudden, this shows up, and it's catastrophic for them. Those kinds of patients, I have to spend a lot more time counseling what to expect and that this is not uncommon and that these are things that occur. So, you're right. What's going on in that mind is key. As surgeons, as therapists, as doctors, we do have a little bit of room to make an impression, but ultimately, what's going on in their head is the final say. Some of my patients are in there like zombies; they want you to take care of it; they don't want any responsibility for their outcomes. They just want you to fix the problem, and they don't understand their part in it.

Clearly there are two parts of the equation in the horror story scenario; part one belongs to the surgeon, part two belongs to you.

You have no control over the surgeon, except in your choice of which surgeon to employ. You have full control over how you participate in your recovery. Increasingly, the studies show that patients with a positive mindset, proper nutrition, and a commitment (there's that word again) to exercising and working on their rehab rarely find their way into a horror story. So, when considering the surgical fix, a bad outcome is not a matter of the luck of the draw. Fear of a bad outcome should not influence your decision to try to live a pain-free life.

One more comment from the doctors about why all the horror stories and then we'll finish up with comments from a couple of our patients. Dr. Christopher Hills in Jackson, Wyoming, answered my question by talking about the use of surgical intervention for back pain based on what is seen on an MRI. He makes a stunning comment about the difference between a surgical success and a clinical disaster. Personally, I found it very reassuring to know that I, the patient, have so much to do with whether a surgery is either perfect or a disaster. It puts a lot more control in my hands and that made me more confident. I believe it will have the same effect on you. Dr. Hills said:

> You could have an absolute perfectly done surgery, textbook, everyone's high-fiving at the end of the case, "Boy, that couldn't have gone better." **You could have an absolute surgical success and have an absolute clinical failure,** and that could be for many reasons. Again, patient expectations. There's a lot of psychosocial issues that come into this, a lot of factors that can give a clinical failure even though you had a surgical success. Having to bring all those together and have them align is critical, and I think that's something we didn't pay close enough attention to in the past when it comes to spine surgery and such. The horror stories are out there that we all have heard and read about.

Yes, we have. And now we have a better idea of why. No matter if you are preparing for spine surgery, hip surgery or simply recovering for a workplace injury, the emotional toll of those events are considerable. As I pointed out in the beginning of this chapter, fear and denial can be nearly as big a barrier to your full function as a broken bone or surgical incision. With this background we are going to have our surgeons guide you on what you should be alert to when considering the surgical fix as you will learn in the next chapter.

Joy H. had a unique and difficult path to accepting the surgical fix. As you will read, making the decision to take the surgical option was a big, and in her own words, a shocking decision. Joy recalls:

> I did look up online for support groups and things like that. I scoured the Internet for the type of procedure I was going to have. I put in exactly what the surgeon had put down that he was going to do, and it didn't even make sense to me. I was searching online, I made my husband sit with me and watch the gory horrific YouTube surgery, that I don't even know what it was, but it was the closest thing I could find that was what I was having. It was the actual open back surgery, on YouTube. I told my husband, "We have to watch this, I need to be prepared. I have nobody to explain what to expect." His face was in his hands, he was just distraught. He said "I can't watch this anymore because I'm gonna be the one awake while they're doing this to you." I was desperate. The underscore part of that is, I was desperate to know what to expect. Scared out of my mind, I knew I had to do this. It felt like it was life or death, really. But I still would've liked to know what to

> expect out of it all, and no one was there. You know that ream of papers they give you to sign, prior to surgery where you're dealing with all the possible outcomes and it kind of explains them. All the legal forms where you sign your life away, really truly.
>
> This sunny afternoon I remember, right before all this was happening. I sat on the deck, looking at this stack of papers and I just sobbed. I was all by myself. "How am I at 28 years old going through this, by myself? How do none of my friends know what this is like?" There was nobody. It was a hard time, really. I think we had a month or two from when doctor said, "Hey, yes I'll do the surgery" to when he actually got me scheduled in the O.R. The first thing I do is just call my parents and say, "Hey, it's happening!" They were very shocked!

Robert G. probably struggled the longest of everyone at the table. His concerns about not being able to enjoy his retirement in Mexico were due, in part, to the horror stories he had heard. When he finally found his way to people who had accepted the surgical fix and won, he made the commitment to put an end to his suffering. This is how Robert told it:

> It was chronic day and night where I literally was not sleeping well. I'm not one for taking pills and drugs. So, to be honest with you, I just lived through all the years until ultimately the third time it came about, and then I had another injection. I want to say that was probably about two years before my surgery, and that injection lasted about a day and a half, where I had no pain. And

then it just all came back with a vengeance—more acute pain or chronic pain consistently day and night no matter what I did.

I really wanted to hold off until I was going to retire March of this year, trying to hold off, but it just got to the point where when I did go to work, and I'm on my feet 10 to 12 hours every day, I couldn't stand for more than five minutes. I was concerned. Actually, I was more concerned that I wouldn't be able to enjoy my retirement. I wanted to be able to do things on my retirement. And, that was my biggest fear. You know, I put a lot of years in my work and just wanted to enjoy the fruits of my labor. But it got to the point where I wasn't even standing up straight. I was hunched over to one side just to try to alleviate the chronic pain that I was having. I finally went in and had the surgery done because I literally could not be on my feet for more than five minutes without really feeling it and actually putting tears to my eyes sometimes. And it did, trust me. Back pain, to me, is one of the worst things I've ever had in my life. Doing the occupation I did, and I'm a big guy—6 feet 5, 270 pounds—it takes a toll. The back, to me, is the most important . . . I mean, there are a lot of other functional things in your body, but as far as pain, it was just tremendous.

From all the exams that I had and the test results, you know exactly what it was. Degenerative disc disease is just part of it. That, over the long run, I think, is what

> ultimately got me to where it spread worse and worse. When you have the disc starting to go, where the fluids were going up against the spine and actually pinching the spine, I guess ultimately that is where all the pain was coming from. I don't know the exact terminology. I just researched what other people had done, different sites on back surgery at the time. Eventually, surgery was, for me, a no-brainer. I mean, everything that I read up on and researched and saw success stories . . . but, you read a lot of horror stories too. Every human is different.

That is why surgery gets a bad rap and, by extension, why so many people are reluctant to decide to have surgery. Think about how much needless suffering Robert endured because of the fear of a possible bad outcome. None of us, unless we are medical students, have a clear and realistic understanding of what we are facing either in surgery or after a serious injury. One of the biggest missing links in the patient recovery process, and the source of much of the fear, is very large lack of patient education material.

In particular, until I started writing this book I had no idea what the problems were with spine surgery.

The good news now is that progress in minimally invasive surgical techniques, improved technology, and a greater knowledge base for the surgeons has dramatically improved patient outcomes.

My follow-up question to the spine surgeons was, "What makes a good candidate for surgery?" It was remarkable, without my prompting, how often the word *optimized* and *optimal* were present in their comments. There are questions that you can, and should, ask your surgeon to make as sure as you possibly can that you are on track to get the outcome you are hoping for. We've heard the patients' fears about what can happen at the hands of their doctor. Now let's hear the doctors' concerns about what makes a great patient.

6

THE SURGEONS' PERSPECTIVE

You've heard the facts behind the horror stories, and having weighed the pros and cons of surgery, you have decided to put an end to your chronic pain. But, are you a good candidate for surgery in the first place? Along the way of writing this book I learned that people want to get better, they just don't know how. Whether lining up for surgery or recovering from a major injury, all of us are amateur patients. As we are learning, just because your back hurts doesn't mean you need or should have surgery. The most interesting part of the conversation that follows is that you and your surgeon are actually a team working to achieve the same goal: to relieve your suffering and to help you become you again. When I first started thinking about how to be an optimized patient, I only looked at it from the patient's point of view. During the interviews, I found out that the surgeons consider both sides of the equation. There is a surgical outcome and there is a clinical outcome. Simply, there is the surgeons' job (the surgical outcome) and, according to them, there's the patient's job (the clinical outcome) which is the healing part—the patient's part of getting better. There is a lot to learn about what makes an optimized patient from the perspective of the surgeon.

The comments of Dr. Christopher Hills in Jackson Hole, Wyoming, merit repeating. He said, "You could have an absolute perfectly done surgery, textbook, everyone's high-fiving at the end of the case, 'Boy, that couldn't have gone better.' **You could have an absolute surgical success and have an absolute clinical failure**, and that could be for many reasons." What? How does a perfect surgery result in total failure?! The reasons that the surgeons detailed were common to all of their decades of experience. In their own words they explain the role of the surgeon and the critical role of the patient. I am sure you're not going to be surprised to hear that patients who are committed to their recovery, who have the *will to get well* are the ones who have the best results. Pay close attention to the doctors' advice if you want the best possible outcome.

Dr. Branko Skovrlj in New Jersey is the youngest of the doctors I interviewed. That means he is closest to what is current in the field. Remarkably, he and all of the surgeons shared a basic concern about what makes a good candidate and how to achieve the best possible outcome. Dr. Branko said:

> With every one of my patients, I sit down and go through all of their films with them, I explain to them exactly what's going on. They have to be part of this game, because if they don't understand and they're not part of the game, how are they going to do well if they don't know what just happened to them or what they went through? So, I explain everything to them, and

then I explain to them on a live model, "Look, this is what we need to do and this is why we need to do it and this is what the evidence shows." So, I spend thirty, forty-five minutes with every patient who needs surgery, explaining exactly what the problem is, what I need to do, why I'm doing it, and then what they can expect and what the risks are of surgery. Everything has to be covered, and then any other questions they have. For me, it's important that my patient is going into the surgery fully understanding as much as they're capable of. They have to have some level of understanding, because I tell them, "Listen, if you're *not* going into this understanding what's going on, with a positive mindset, and looking forward to getting better, then whatever I do for you is for nothing. You're not gonna get better."

Dr. Khurana talks in detail about what happened to me. I was not the perfect patient nor particularly typical, but how he chronicles my case is right at the heart of the surgeon's perspective. Be alert to the assessment he makes of my actual injury as well as the assessment of my mental attitude. Interestingly enough, none of this was really discussed when I came to him as a patient. This is not to say he didn't fully inform me about the procedure and the available options. He was very thorough about that. But, what I found fascinating was how he sized me up as a patient. It is right in line with what Dr. Hills and Dr. Branko have said. It's not just about what is happening in your back. There are many considerations that surgeons use to evaluate who will benefit from surgery.

As a patient, or prospective patient, their insights are part of the education you need to prepare for the best possible outcome.

Dr. Justin Saliman observed a number of life-style and attitude realities that he considers when assessing a patient's chances of a good outcome from surgery. Dr. Saliman said with some concern,

> You actually can live longer if you're doing a lot of these mind/body things like meditation and healthy diet. So, there's no question that those are going to improve a patient's ability to, first of all, not get sick in the first place, and then recover once they are sick or injured. Certainly, for big procedures like spine procedures and joint replacements, the patient's makeup does make a big difference in terms of their likelihood to do things like get infected or their ability to heal quickly. Patients who are severely diabetic, there's very good evidence, do not heal as well after spine, hip, or joint replacement. Same with body mass index. So, obese patients tend to not heal as well, like literally the cells in your body when you're diabetic, for example, just don't heal as quickly. A lot of type 2 diabetes has to do with diet and exercise. If you can affect that pre-operatively and maintain it post-operatively, you're more likely to heal faster and more fully, which basically affects your outcome.

When I asked Dr. Vermon Esplin tell me what a patient who is likely to recovery looks like when he or she is sitting across the table from him. Dr. Esplin replied,

> That looks like somebody who comes in who basically is asking a number of questions, who's already

> checked around, they know what the options are, they know that it's going to take a certain amount of time and what to expect. The ones that are asking questions and are already physically good condition whose history is that they've had challenges and have overcome them and managed through them, even though they may have had some complication along the way, they still were very positive and still going to face the challenges no matter what came their way, as opposed to the middle ground where people come in, and you tell them what you've got to do, and that's all they want to hear, they don't want to hear about the other stuff or what to expect. But people who are motivated, who have a plan, who have a reason, they want to get better by this date, or they have a forward-thinking plan of what the outcome is going to be and what the rehab is going to take and what their part in it is going to be.

Dr. Khurana's comments began in response to my question, "Tell me what a surgeon is looking for as they assess whether or not that person is a good candidate for surgery?" Dr. Khurana replied specifically using my experience as an example,

> When we looked at your imaging, I was struck by how profound the degeneration in your back was at the levels causing the problem.
>
> So, first of all, the diagnosis when I was evaluating you, was based on the combination of the symptoms that you had, in addition to the progression, your own acknowledged progression of those symptoms, as

> it related to your gait dysfunction, and atrophy of the calves, and a lot of the bladder dysfunction and so forth, coupled with the structural findings. As you recalled, I thought it would take probably four to four and a half hours, and it ended up taking probably 30% longer, just because of the magnitude and the intensity of your nerve compression. And the one thing that struck me pretty intensely was the sheer magnitude of nerve compression at L4/5 that you had. It was basically to the point where the nerves were constricted from a normal configuration of up to two centimeters and it was constricted really, down to about three to four millimeters. And so, it just really required a lot of picking away of those tissues which had been calcified and compressed and wrapped around your nerve roots.
>
> I remember when I saw you in the hospital, I think I told you something to the effect of, "You'll feel like you got hit by a Mack truck" and you said something to the effect of, "Yeah I feel like I got hit by a Mack truck and more."

I nodded remembering, "Yeah, I was planning to get hit by a bus, but it was actually a Mack truck." I recall you also said that you hadn't seen that much nerve damage in a back in anyone who wasn't already in a wheelchair. And you were sort of amazed that I was still actually walking or not in a wheelchair already.

Dr. Khurana continued,

> Over a 15-year career so far, you really get to see the variation of anatomy and pathology and different

degrees of presentation. In the lumbar spine, there's a little bit more flexibility in your degree of compression before it causes complete neurological injury. So just to be clear, your spinal cord starts in your brain and it ends at about the level of your belly button, that's the actual substance and the continuation of, actually, your brain. But the spinal cord actually has nerve roots that come off of it at multiple segments, particularly in the last inch or two of the spinal cord. And those little branches form nerve roots that come out to your lumbar spine, and they're held by the lumbar spinal sack; it holds all the nerve roots which are kind of the hair that comes off the spinal cord. And so, because there are a bunch of, essentially, spaghetti strings in a water balloon, if you will, for a simplistic way to do it, it requires an extraordinary amount of compression to cause multiple nerve roots to be injured. It would require extraordinary, chronic, and severe compression to cause frank paralysis.

But, in cases like yours where you had, actually atrophy of the calves, and dysfunction of your gastrox and calf muscles, it was the same point of explanation. The explanation was the most inner nerve roots at that level, the sacral nerve roots, were actually injured by simple ischemia. They had no ability for the small vessels to squeeze oxygen into those nerve roots because they were compressed so severely in the central part of the spinal sack. So, when you look at the bell curve and where you

> were relative to a lot of folks, it was way on the tail end of the bell curve. It was just extraordinary. Just the fact that you were able to even have that degree of function that you had when you saw me was more of a testament to yourself than it was to the condition. You were able to kind of schlonk through despite that problem.

Schlonk is a highly technical medical term for limping around. A very funny story about that. I was on my way into a Starbucks. There is a fellow with a paper cup in his hand asking customers for money as they enter the store. He sees me coming and says, "Hey, I see you've got a bum leg too." It stunned me to think my limp was that obvious. Without thinking I said, "Hey, thanks for pointing that out for everyone! Really." As if I wasn't feeling bad enough about the hangover nerve damage that was still healing after the surgery.

I asked Dr. Branko what defines a patient as a good candidate for surgery? It seemed to me that once you dig into it, there are a lot of factors that figure into the horror stories. Dr. Branko squarely addressed the patient's role, your role in a great outcome. Dr. Branko thought about it a second. Choosing his words carefully, he said:

> I tell my patients, straight, up-front. I tell them that, **"Look, before you go into surgery, you have to think about what you're getting into."** And I tell them, "Listen, you will not do well unless you are positive about this surgery." Meaning that you know that after surgery, you will get better, because you will work on it. And it takes some people a couple days, some people a couple

weeks, some people a couple months to come to grips with what they're about to get into. And somebody needs to plant that seed into them early, that your positive mindset and your will, like a sheer will, to get better, is going to have to be part of this whole process. And I think if they enter the surgery with this kind of mindset, one, they're going to do better, two, they're probably going to have less pain, and three, they're probably going to need less narcotics.

But this is a very macho society and a lot of guys don't want to hear this stuff. Like "Oh, you know, I'm not a girl." I've had some patients tell me that. It's like, "Oh, come on, I'm not like a girl here. I'm a guy, a big guy, I know what to do." I always tell my patients when I do the ALIF procedure—where we go in through the front—and they ask me, "How long am I gonna be in the hospital?" I say, "You're a guy. You're probably going to be in the hospital for two days. If you're a woman, you probably go home the next day because women deal with pain much better." And they all laugh.

Harvey, you got the shish kabob and you're doing great! Every time you have a surgery, no matter how minimally invasive it is, there's always a chance of a complication. As long as you have a good outcome at the end, it doesn't matter if you have three approaches or thirty-three approaches. It doesn't matter. Look, unless somebody butchers you, and there are plenty of guys who can do that surgery, the majority of people are

> going to do it correctly. It doesn't have to be done so that it looks textbook, the images afterwards. As long as it achieves the goal it was supposed to achieve, that part is done. But, the most important part is the patient's mindset, for me. It's their attitude and how much are they willing to get better. How positive they are. How much are they willing to push to get better.

It was interesting to me that our role, the patients' role, kept surfacing in the comments by the doctors. Surgeons see the part they play in a patient's effort to get well in a very specific way. This was especially evident in the viewpoint as we just heard from Dr. Branko. He continues:

> Because there's another problem in this particular culture. In Croatia, where I'm from, people pretty much do everything they can to not have surgery. Or, if they have to have surgery, they do exactly what you're talking about right now. They really try to prepare for it, but what I'm seeing here is that a lot of people feel like "Yeah. Let's do surgery," but they don't really know what they're getting into.

Dr. Hills from Jackson, Wyoming, is particularly interesting in that his comments begin in the clinical findings–how the imaging lines up with his exam. He, like Dr. Branko and Dr. Khurana, turns to an assessment of the patient's mindset. I think in the simplest terms they all look back to the beginning of this book. They are all underlining the importance of the patient's "commitment" and their will to get well. Dr. Hills said:

> Yes. I think there are numerous factors or what you would call multifactorial. Number one, they have to have appropriate diagnosis with imaging that corresponds to their clinical findings, that is there are many people that have significant pathology throughout their spine, and their pain may not be associated to their MRI imaging or what diagnosis is made from an MRI imaging. It's their clinical exam correlating to their MRI findings. Number two, they should be in relatively good health and optimized, as you say. Number three, surgical expectations are paramount in this decision. If you have unrealistic expectations then that's where we fall short many times in spine surgery, because we're unable to meet those expectations, or the surgeon has different surgical expectations than the patient does. Those have to coincide, and we have to be on the same playing field when it comes to what the surgical expectation is and the goals are of the procedure. When all those things align then I feel the patient is a good surgical candidate to try to have the best outcome possible.

I wondered whether or not there were times when, from a surgeon's perspective, they are sitting across from a patient who they actually evaluate as not a good candidate for surgery. Dr. Hills continued,

> Well, again, that could be multifactorial. Number one, secondary intention. We know many times, like with Workman's Compensation or litigation, there are some secondary motives to wanting spine surgery.

> Number two, if they're not optimized, if they have significant comorbidities [multiple health issues], then the risk factors outweigh the benefits of the procedure, especially if it's an elective surgery. Number three, often there are unrealistic expectations. Can we guarantee we can get all patients back to high-functioning levels with certain spine procedures? We can't guarantee that many times. If surgical expectations are beyond a realistic goal, then that person is not a good candidate.

Considering that guideline, I might have been considered not a good candidate. I pointed that out to Dr. Hills this way, "That's really funny. I'm going to chime in that my doctor thought that it would be 18 months until I had full use of my calves, and stuff, again. I was almost wheelchair bound. Actually, it's taken four years for me to recover full function. I'm in my 60s and I'm in pretty darn good shape. I'm writing an optimized book because I'm pretty optimized. If my expectation had been four years to regain full function perhaps I wouldn't have done it, so it's kind of a mixed bag."

We agreed that is a real consideration. It really is a conundrum. On the one hand you want to have hope that you can recover. On the other hand, you want your surgeon to give you the facts so you can together develop a realistic expectation. If Dr. Khurana and I had guessed it would take four years for my full recovery, would I have done it? Probably. With the understanding that, just like Joy H., I would have expected to beat the odds and recover sooner than later. Am I glad I committed to surgery? Absolutely. With regard to a surgeon painting a rosy picture, I think they should give us a look at the best possible outcome even if there is a chance we might not get the result we hoped for. What is the axiom in basketball? 100% you are going to miss the shot you never take. I took the chance that Dr. Khurana would make the shot, and he did.

I suggested to Dr. Hills that some of the people who are reading this book may not have yet walked into a spine surgeon's office and have no idea exactly what spine surgeons do. He said he would try to make it simple for patients reading this book to have some context. Dr. Hills explained:

> So, in probably simplest terms available in spine surgery, we do two things. One is a decompression, that is taking pressure off the spinal cord, the nerve roots, or the spinal elements in some form or fashion. So, just creating more room for the spinal cord elements. On the other hand, there are times where we do fusions where you take away motion from a segment of the spine, one or multiple segments of the spine. There are some patients who are indicated for just decompression. There are some who are clearly indicated for fusion. There is some gray area in between those two.
>
> Now, the main indications for a fusion are instability. That is, if you have a slippage of one bone on the other. Scoliosis is a form of instability. You have things such as fractures and tumors that can cause instability. Those are clear indications for fusion. Part of the fusion is a decompression, whether it's what we call direct where you go in and manually open up the spinal canal, or the foramen, where the nerves exit out. The other method

> is indirect, relying on the implants to do some of that work for you. There are patients who do not have frank instability that many times can have an equal, or better, outcome with just a decompression. You do not need to do the fusion, which is the larger of the two procedures, where it's a bigger recovery. Again, there is some gray area there where someone might have some micro-instability, if you will, that when you do a decompression it could potentially lead to further instability down the road as a part of their degenerative process that was also occurring or, in addition, the surgical procedure itself can lead to some slight instability. There is a gray area there, and that's kind of where the devil is in the details of trying to look ahead and prognosticate who is going to fall into that gray area and try to make a decision on the factors that are present.

As I mentioned earlier, Dr. Branko is among the spine surgeons who come to the operating room without a lot of history or investment in traditional methodology. He looks back at the mistakes of the past without being part of the era of surgeons who created the outcomes that concern every spine patient. Dr. Branko gave this perspective:

> I did neurosurgery training for seven years and I've been out in my own practice for two years. So, in total, I've been in this thing for nine years. Every year, new stuff comes out, and there's a better understanding of things. When the patients go out there and look for a surgeon, or they go and get an opinion, they can go

> see somebody who just came out of training recently, somebody who is mid-career, or somebody who's been practicing for twenty, twenty-five years. Every one of these guys is going to see things in different perspectives, because this whole field of spine surgery has just been evolving so rapidly. So, the guys who have been doing things for twenty, twenty-five years, they're doing them the way they've been trained way back when. And the fields have really changed massively since then. So, that's why you can go to three different guys and they'll all give you different opinions. Vastly different opinions, meaning one will say, "Oh, you may only need a laminectomy, meaning removing bone around the nerve, taking pressure off the nerve." Where another guy will tell you, "Oh, I think you need a fusion, as well," meaning we have to fuse your spine together. And then as soon as the patient hears the word *fusion*, they get scared, because fusion has a bad reputation.

We also discussed what the physical therapists said about alternatives to surgery and when it's time to see the surgeon. So, when is it time to see the surgeon from the surgeon's perspective? Dr. Branko went on,

> So, that's an excellent question and I don't think there is a specific answer for that. Every patient, we see totally different problems. What I mean by that is that you can have ten patients come in who have, let's say, cervical disc herniation, and they have compression on the nerve and they need some sort of surgery. Well, every

> single one of these patients is going to have a different anatomy, a different alignment of the spine, different things going on at different discs above and below. All that stuff needs to be put into perspective when you decide what you are planning to do for them. Because if you don't look into all these things, you're predisposing this patient to have problems down the road where they may do well for six months to a year, and then other problems may start from what you did or from what you didn't do. And the, the pain starts again and then they may need another surgery and here comes the bad outcome. They're not happy, they're not satisfied, they thought this was going to be a one-time deal; they were going to be better. Well, now they're back, and somebody tells them, "You may need more surgery. Things broke down. Your spine is breaking down." So, all these things . . . everybody's so different. So, what is the right reason to do spine surgery is a difficult answer.

Dr. Sanjay Khurana wanted to make sure that he was clear from the surgeon's perspective. He added:

> There are just a couple things on the surgical end that will optimize you as a patient. There are many things on your side that will optimize you as a patient. So, from the standpoint of a surgeon's perspective of what makes a patient a good candidate, there's really, let's just say three things, and I think that they will be echoed on the patient's side as well. But, from a surgical indication's standpoint, you have to be extraordinarily

> confident that the imaging and the findings that you see are directly correlated to the symptoms that you have. So that's my end. That's my duty to a patient, just to make that correlation. That's why the schooling is so long—that's why with practice over time you get better at identifying these patterns.

When coming from the spine surgeons, the core of what *The Optimized Patient* is all about has a little bit of a different spin. So, **if this is what surgeons think makes for a successful surgery and a great patient recovery, let's pay very close attention.** A final observation from Dr. Hills:

> It starts before surgery, and it's all about education. You need to know what your options are. You need to do everything you can preoperatively, because most of the time these are not emergency procedures, and there are many things you can do conservatively. You need to maximize those to be able to have the best—even surgical—outcome, if you get to that point. Most of these conditions can be treated conservatively, so maximize those things. It comes to this: weight control, appropriate nutrition, activity. We know that bed rest is not the best case for most spine conditions. We want to keep you active with non-impact aerobic conditioning, core strengthening, and just overall good mental health state is critical when it comes to conditions of the spine.

Those are the pillars of becoming an optimized patient and having the best possible outcome from your spine surgery, or as we learned from my friend Adam Rodman, to recover from any kind of surgery.

Thank you, Dr. Hills for providing a perfect summary to the surgeon's perspective and a relevant introduction to Chapter 7, "Why Optimize?" Let's take a closer look at why I think every patient planning any kind of surgery should optimize. Although this book is focused on spine surgery, my screenwriter friend Adam Rodman, who knew about *The Optimized Patient* concept, adopted it before surgery for his septum. You'll learn more about his story in Chapter 12, "Becoming You Again."

Another friend of mine prepared for prostate surgery after observing my outcome and also had a recovery that was, according to his doctor, dramatically better than most—if not all. Subsequently, the approach I am detailing in this book helped me enjoy a remarkable recovery from my prostate surgery and a partial knee replacement. As I said, this is not a book about science and testing. It's a book about patient experience. Those close to me watched me and they believed, "If he can optimize, I can optimize." They did optimize and so can you.

7

WHY OPTIMIZE?

The more precise question is what will it take to get well, to be me again? Very few people, other than medical professionals, even understand how human beings get better. Is it the cast that heals your arm or is it your arm that heals your arm? Right, your body is programmed to heal. You don't really have to think your body into healing a wound or clearing up a bruise, it just does it—when the conditions are right. Most patients approaching any kind of surgery feel that the surgeon is going to do the work and they are just along for the ride. My body is going to do what my body is programmed to do, right? Well, kinda. As we heard in the "Surgeon's Perspective," there is a surgical outcome and a clinical outcome. The clinical outcome is the one in your control. Helping your body to fully recover pain-free function is the very definition of a clinical success and the reason why anyone preparing for spine surgery should know how to optimize.

In Chapter 4, "What Are My Options?" Physical Therapist, Solomon Joseph, opened the door to our understanding about the prehab benefits of aqua therapy. If you recall, he said if you walked around in a swimming pool in chest-high water an hour a day, three times a week for a couple of months before surgery, one of two things would happen: 1) you might not need surgery or 2) your chance of a full recovery would be greatly enhanced. It's point 2 that we will focus on in this chapter.

Would you be interested in optimizing if you knew that it would improve your chances for a full recovery?

Having had three spine surgeries I am fairly confident that the answer is, "Which way is the pool?" My investigation into aqua therapy began with a tip from Bill Walton. Because of our conversation, I asked my physical therapists if Bill knew what the heck he was talking about. Sure enough, he was right on target.

But, don't take my, or Bill's, word for it. Listen to Solomon Joseph, Physical Therapist and Aqua Therapy specialist at Advanced Orthopedic Physical Therapy in Long Beach, California. Solomon says:

> The biggest benefit I find to Aqua Therapy is the buoyancy when you get in the water—it unloads your system. It takes a lot of pressure off your muscles and usually, when you're rehabbing, (prehabbing or rehabbing) spinal injuries and surgeries, your muscles are very weak, and for them to move under stress of your body weight, it's a lot more challenging. So, getting in the water takes a lot of pressure off the muscles. It allows them to do a lot more movement and exercise with a lot less stress. That being said, the movement of the joints in your spine or out in your lower extremities, need to

be controlled as well, and when you get in the water, it actually slows down motions quite a bit. Motion is very effective for rehabbing because the faster your spine moves, your joints move, the faster your muscles have to react to the motion of these joints.

In the seven years I have struggled with and overcome disabling back pain that is the single best and most absolutely on the mark piece of advice that I came across.

Solomon went on to say,

> The water gets chest-high and that takes about 70 percent to 80 percent of the weight off. So, if you weigh 200 pounds at chest height you're pretty much weighing 40 to 50 pounds. And you could lose a few pounds with exercise. So, when you're standing and doing these functional exercises in the pool, it translates a lot easier on land once you get stronger. So, they can get in there and have pain be their guide, as far as moving and jumping around and exercising and building strength while they're unloaded in the water system.

Solomon explained the term "unloading" for clarity:

> That is where they actually strap a harness around your waist, around your chest, and lift part of your body weight up overhead and that takes a lot of pressure off your lower extremities and off your spine. So, you can exercise or decrease the amount of pressure on your spine. Very similar to when you get into the pool and you feel like you are unloading in your system, you feel

> lighter on your feet, lighter on your muscles and everything else.

That makes all the sense in the world. Put your body in a nearly zero gravity environment in the water and then use the water like a giant resistance device. You unload and condition at the same time as you do the very simple work of just walking in chest-high water around the pool. I wish I had known that before my first surgery. I took a little different, harder, approach in the gym.

Once I had made the commitment and set a date, I knew I was going to get hit by a bus on December 22nd. Not literally, of course, but figuratively. I was going to wake up after surgery with steel in my back (see x-ray image on book cover) and incisions in three places on my midsection. So, at 64, I hunkered down and made the commitment to do the weight training needed to get me in optimal shape. If I knew then what I know now, I would have certainly preferred to walk around a pool for an hour rather than laboring through challenging, exhausting, and sometimes painful weight training. By the way, in my aqua therapy class were people recovering from knee, hip and shoulder injuries, many of them had not had surgery.

I also knew that my range of motion was going to be much diminished. It seemed to me that yoga would also be a great preparatory regimen. When I discussed my prehab ideas with Dr. Khurana he asked me the following questions. "Can you touch your toes?" I said, "Sure, no problem." He continued, as if to challenge me, "Can you put your palms on the floor?" I proudly said, "You betcha!" As serious as a heart attack he grimly said, "Don't ever do that again." After I stopped laughing he said, "No. Really.

Don't ever do that again. That kind of hyperextension can do more harm than good." I recount that story to make sure that you don't overdo it in whatever conditioning plan suits you for whatever your injury is, check with your doctor. Challenge yourself, get ready for the hit, but do not go nuts.

Cardio conditioning is also very important. Remember, you are going to be fairly sedentary for a little bit during the early days of your recovery. The physical therapists were particularly keen on prehab. Trying to master the movements essential to your recovery is very challenging after surgery. Ironically, the first time most patients see the physical therapist is when they come limping in the door in a back brace or with a walker or both and then they have to learn a whole set of completely unfamiliar movements. Doesn't it make sense to optimize with those movements *before* surgery so on top of being physically challenged you are not also insecure and nervous about your rehab plan? I think it makes all the sense in the world, but it is rarely done.

Fortunately, new thinking is emerging with advocacy both from the surgeons and the physical therapists. The hope is to get the insurance companies on board for an optimized plan that will help patients get better faster and stay better longer. Remember the biggest issue we heard from the spine surgeons was that they were doing excellent surgery and total clinical failures were occurring because the patient didn't do what was essential to properly and fully recover function.

Dr. Branko leaned in on this at the 30,000 foot view. Dr. Branko said:

> People want instantaneous results. They don't want any involvement. So, just like you said, there's no magic wand. We're here to facilitate the healing. We're here to put your body into a place where you can take over and heal it, but a lot of patients, they just want to come in and out, be fixed, and move on to doing what they were doing before, which leads to the problem of not taking care of themselves.

They haven't yet realized they are going to get hit by a bus, and they need to prepare. Remember, at the beginning of the book I said it's a commitment. Dr. Branko, without my prompting, said something very similar from a surgeon's point of view:

> Well, obviously, the way I would put it to the patient is, "Listen, you obviously want to put your body into a state where it's going to be capable of healing itself. And you need to load up your body with the nutrients and the vitamins and the minerals and put it in that kind of state where everything that I'm going to do to your back, which is a big surgery, you're going to be able to heal from it within a certain time span so that you don't develop chronic issues afterwards. And the nutrition is going to be extremely important in that, because if you don't have the building blocks to rebuild what I helped you create here, and to heal it, you may have problems. If you have delayed healing, wound issues, or if you don't heal within a certain period of time, you may enter into this kind of inflammatory condition and you

may endure pain for longer periods of time." **Nutrition is a key for your part of the surgery, for sure.**

Dr. Branko continued,

> Activity has a lot to do with it. How healthy you were or how active you were before surgery has a big, big impact on how well you're going to do after surgery. I'll tell you this, it only took me maybe a couple surgeries into my residency to realize who the smokers are and who are not. I don't even have to see you before your surgery. I can come into your surgery when you're fully draped, and I can make a skin incision and I can within five seconds tell if you're a smoker or not. Just from looking at your tissue. Everything is thinned out; you can just tell, immediately. You know it, straight away. So, the people who take care of their bodies, their bodies are going to respond much better to this insult that we create, and they're going to do much better versus those people who never did any exercise before, whose body is just kinda getting by. Those who don't eat well, the guys who smoke, they're already at the limit. They don't have any reserves. So, now you put them through surgery, they're struggling big time to get back.

If your surgeon hasn't already told you all of that, now you have been told.

Dr. Hills of Jackson, Wyoming, was equally emphatic about your role in the best outcome. He was very strong on education and preparation. Dr. Hills explained:

> I think pre-operatively it takes many visits with a physician, with the providers, outlining postoperatively how they're going to work on this post rehab, and then things such as education classes with the hospital, the physician, so you know exactly what's going to take place once the day of the procedure is performed, and then thereafter, so that there are no surprises. They know exactly what they're walking into, and when everyone's on the same playing field with the same expectations, then I think that's where everyone's going to have the best outcomes possible.

I said, "I will assert in the book that it's a commitment on the part of the patient to get involved in his own recovery. How would you underline that?

Dr. Hills quickly answered, "I'd double underline it. It's all about the patient. It really is." If the Optimized Patient is about anything it is about patient education. I have often joked on television Interviews that I was absent the day they taught Surgery Recovery 101. That lack of knowing is a problem for each and every patient facing surgery or recovery from a major Injury. None of us have been here before. None of us know the road ahead. I think Bill Walton said it best, "You want a coach who has been to the place you want to go." That is who Bill was for me and who Nathan Quarry was for Doug Amend. A guide, a coach a teacher showing us the way to a full recovery.

My surgeon, Dr. Khurana, and his colleagues have a definite point of view on what I call optimizing and what he calls pre-habilitation. You may see the genesis of the optimized patient concept in his comments. Dr. Khurana believes:

> From a functional standpoint, from a patient, just from a nuts and bolts perspective of getting patients to the finish line, one thing that I started subscribing at the behest of a lot of physical therapists was this concept called pre-habilitation. Pre-habilitation is really like training for a marathon. If you're going to do a race, or you're going to undertake a traumatic event like a surgery, you really want to build your core, your nerves, even your physiological reserve so when you do have surgery, you're more likely to recover more smoothly. And that's something I've only relatively recently been adding to the surgical courses is this concept of pre-habilitation.
>
> And pre-habilitation can really take many different forms. Some people will go to a chiropractor where that will be their form of pre-habilitation. Others will go to physical therapy and that will be their form of pre-habilitation. Part of me says it's just a way of naming a non-operative treatment course prior to surgery, but I think the label of pre-habilitation really gives the patient a sense of their goal of therapy may not be a solution in and of itself, but may be part of the solution so that it will help expedite recovery post-surgery. And so that's something I'm actively pursuing with regional physical therapists—developing programs to have that concept of pre-habilitation and hopefully even get buy-in by the insurers that this is a doable and reasonable part of the

commitment by an insurance company to optimize patient outcomes.

Dr. Khurana mentions the physical therapists and his belief that better preparation with their help makes for better outcomes. Let's hear how the physical therapists see their role in the optimized patient approach.

Physical Therapist, Patti Sogaard, was happy to hear Dr. Khurana's point of view. She added:

> I usually do not see spine patients for prehab, I will see patients who will rehab to try to avoid surgery, rather than prehab if it's the spine. So, an MD refers a patient for prehab if there's a traumatic injury, causing swelling or decreased joint function in mobility. **Studies have shown if a patient goes into surgery with close to a healthy joint, as close as possible, then recovery afterwards is easier and more likely to be successful.** Plus, it also gives the patient some education on post-surgical recovery, such as what to expect; for instance, if patients are using an assisted device they then know how to use it before they go in rather than afterwards. Again, prehab helps to decrease pain and stiffness before going into surgery, but prehab also educates the patient on what to expect after surgery. I think unreal expectations can actually make recovery more difficult for the patient.

I had never heard the word "prehab" while preparing for surgery. It's a relatively new idea as it relates to improved surgical outcomes. All I was after was to get optimized before I got hit by the bus. I know that's not very scientific or sanitary, but it sure is accurate. I asked Patti, "So you see prehab as a conversation with a physical therapist that will help patients understand what lies ahead on the road?"

Patti helped expand my understanding of prehab and how it relates to becoming optimized. Patti explained:

> I think it's a very important aspect of it, especially if they have a lot of pain and tightness. But we will also be able to decrease some of the pain and inflammation of other joints which can also make rehab afterwards easier. **The patient needs to become educated on injury so they have a better understanding of what to realistically expect from their outcome.** I expect compliance, listening to the doctors and physical therapists because they are the ones who are educated and experienced in proper recovery. The MDs (doctors) and the PTs (physical therapists) are only part of the recovery; if patients do not do their part, they won't have the best recovery possible. I think it's very difficult for a patient to get a full, good, healthy outcome without a proper diagnosis of what your limitations really are; you want to be able to diagnose the body's range of motion, limitations, and weaknesses. People get very used to how they're walking, how they feel, and after a while it's habit, so they actually don't even see what some of their limitations are. So, they don't understand how to fully recover from those limitations.

I told Patti, "What I've learned from working with you is that there is a pace that's too much and it's counterproductive, and there is a pace and sequence to a physical therapist's method." We went on to discuss the importance of a measured and well thought out plan for recovery. We will talk a lot about that in Chapter 9, "Win or Lose in Rehab."

Patti followed up:

> I think when a patient starts with a healthy spine, they are taught exercises and how to strengthen a healthy spine. They're not really taught how to or ever had the experience of doing very limited exercises that won't damage their tissues. They're only used to healthy tissue. But what they've done most likely was leading up to this injury, so it was damaging from the start. Now, after injury or surgery, somebody has to guide them through the weakened tissue, the tight tissue, the vulnerable tissue, the nerve pain, and you really need an educated physical therapist to properly retrain a person to know how to gain strength without just continuing to damage.

Long before I had my first thought about writing a book about how to prepare for, survive, and recover from surgery, our group of patients were already optimizing in their own way without even knowing it or planning to do so. When I invited Lucio, Joy, Robert, Linda, and Doug to contribute to the book and told them the premise, they were thrilled to help codify a protocol for the patients yet to come. Despite the fact that they had done exactly what they needed to do to recover fully, they all wished that there had been a book to follow. None of us, and I speak for the group, would have left our best recovery to chance or dumb luck if there had been a book on how to optimize. Now the patients will have their say, what did they actually do and what was the outcome?

Our mortgage banker/mountain climber Doug Amend put it this way:

> The interesting thing was, and you kind of alluded to it in our first conversation, was that if people had the opportunity to schedule a surgery out like you did, with the express intent of getting themselves in better shape before surgery, that they would reap the benefits during recovery by doing that. I just happened to have used a three or four month program prior to surgery to improve my health, cardio, all this other stuff, and yes, I can absolutely attest that I believe I healed better because of it.

Dumb luck and great timing. It seemed to be a recurrent theme as the conversation continued. Homemaker, Linda B., made her own good luck. I asked her if she could recall making an effort to get ready for her surgery. I am not calling what she did optimizing, because the idea had not yet been established. But, optimizing is exactly what she did. Linda said:

> I walked every day. I have a lot of hills around my house, and I visualized building my heart stronger for the surgery. Definitely, I pushed myself to continue walking because I wanted to be stronger for the surgery. I gave up drinking too. I'm not a big drinker. I like wine, but I didn't drink for about a two-year period. I'd say

> maybe six months before the surgery and then like after because I felt I wanted to do everything that I could to make my bones feel better. So, I ate more greens, anything that I thought would help my body mend faster. This surgery was gonna put me back quite a bit and I needed to do everything on my part and in my power to participate in making my healing better. So yeah, if there was something that I could do and if it was as simple as not having a glass of wine or eating more vegetables or going for that walk, I definitely did it.

Linda summarizes the entire optimized patient concept perfectly:

"I needed to do everything on my part and in my power to participate in making my healing better."

There it is in a nutshell. That's the heart of getting optimized—to get better faster and stay better longer.

We have already learned that our entrepreneur and restaurateur, Lucio D., is a very physically fit and active fellow. What we are about to find out now is that there's a little bit of the Boy Scout in him as well. Lucio talked to his doctor about his blood work and made a conscious commitment to be prepared. Lucio recalled it saying:

> Let me get myself at a point where I'm just a perfect candidate to go under the knife. And that's me, though. I'm that type of person that goes, okay, I'm getting ready to do something, let me really get prepared, as much as I can. And I did that. As soon as I got the blood test back,

> I was told, "Looks like everything's good, you just need to cut back on stress." And that was really the only thing we talked about, was just don't get stressed out about this stuff. But, I already had a decent diet. I think I cut back on eating glutens at that point. I wanted to stay at a certain level. No drinking whatsoever, no alcohol, zero. Even the wine, none of that, just totally stopped that. And I decided to take it a little healthier—a lot more vegetables, not a lot of meat, keep the digestive system moving regularly.
>
> These are the things that kind of went through my mind, but I'm a preparer. I was a Boy Scout when I was younger, so I always try to prepare myself. And maybe that's what some people need to hear. "Hey, by the way, now that you've got your blood test and they tell you where you're at, you need to cut back on sugar because you've got high blood sugar, you need to take it down. You need to work on that. If your A1C is up, you need to bring that down because you're going to go under the knife. You want your heart not to have to struggle, and your breathing not to have to struggle when you're under the knife. These people are already doing a surgery on you. You want to make sure that you're making it as easy as possible for them. And more importantly, Lucio, to make the surgery and recovery as easy as possible on you."

We will close this chapter with our violinist, Joy H. It is important to note that some of the methods she tried before surgery paid dividends after surgery as well. That is another core concept of *The Optimized Patient*; **the physical and mental work you do before surgery will hasten the day of your full recovery.** Again, all of the patients at the table never heard about the optimized strategy until we started talking about it. Joy H. recounted her journey this way:

> It didn't really dawn on me to plan ahead and be strategic about optimizing my health in order to go through surgery well. What I was trying to do initially was to just control pain—a diet to control pain, because no one was going to do a surgery on me. That was how it all began. But I think it ended up paying off, because what you're willing to try before, it illustrates your willingness to try anything later to heal from a surgery. It did end up paying off, and I learned some things. Calling anything I did a strategy would be a stretch. I pretty much stuck with what I'd done so far, in life, which is to stay thin and stay moving. I ate balanced, kept moving with my life. Because my pain was still present, it was as bad as ever, so it wasn't like I could do more. I couldn't suddenly become a gym rat. That was still hindering me, but I didn't alter anything really dramatically. Someone recommended some breathing, practical breathing exercises, just for pain management prior to my surgery. That was something I did learn on my own . . . just breathing from YouTube videos and things like that.
>
> The breathing for healing and pain management, that was something new that I'd never gotten into, and I think was pretty awesome. It wasn't a cure for all my

> pain, obviously, but it was a neat way to mentally get myself in a position to take a moment and just breathe. I don't know, I don't want it to sound like it was a spiritual endeavor, definitely not. I know it can be for some people, like with the yoga thing. For me, it was just strictly flooding my veins with oxygen. That and the healing practice of that. I thought that was really helpful. If there's anything I added, it would've been that: learning to breathe deeply to control intense pain. That really came in handy afterwards as well because I couldn't get comfortable.

Every one of the patients, doctors, and physical therapists not only agree with the preparatory concept of *The Optimized Patient*, they were also disappointed that they had no guide like this book to help them. As Joy H. said, she had no "strategy." None of us did. But, now you should be beginning to understand and appreciate how important an optimizing strategy really is. And now the big day is on the calendar. You have heard a lot about the need to prepare. Unlike those of us sharing our experiences in this book, you are going to know what to ask your surgeon *before* your surgery. This is yet another key element of the plan to optimize.

8

KNOW WHAT TO ASK . . . BEFORE

There is great comfort in replacing fear with facts. For me, having spine surgery was like going to a foreign country. There was a whole new language to learn and a lot of very unfamiliar territory. If you have ever planned a trip overseas, you know the general process of preparing to experience something entirely different. I have to admit, I am a lot better at planning trips and knowing what I want to do before traveling than I was at planning for surgery and the subsequent recovery. I know how to travel. I knew nothing about my spine before my first surgery. If you are recovering from a major injury I am confident that you are doing a lot of reading about how to regain full function and much of sounds like a foreign language. True to the travel analogy, my second surgery and the third were a lot less challenging because I had already learned the language and the road map. With the new knowledge gained from my first surgery I recall having many questions as I prepared for my second surgery, "Shouldn't I be...? Would it help if I ...?

Wouldn't it be better if we ..." Knowing what to ask before your surgery is key to the optimized patient strategy.

Even though the surgeons have a duty to keep you properly informed, they really don't have the ability to spend hours to address all of the fears that patients considering or preparing for surgery may have. All of us gathered at this table tried to find facts on the Internet. As we alluded to earlier, much of the information on the Internet is guaranteed to scare the pants off of you, to put it politely! (I have no doubt you will look anyway. I did and so did everyone else.) The optimized approach takes into account many factors that prepare you for a successful outcome. Key to that success, in the opinion of the surgeons, physical therapists and patients, is education and a positive mental attitude. Education usually brings to mind a very dry and boring experience of reviewing charts and data. You won't find that here. The most important part of your education is grasping and understanding the details of what your journey is going to entail and how to have your mind in the right place to have the most positive experience possible. The first question to ask yourself *before* they roll you in the operating room is, **"Is my head on straight and am I ready to do the hard work of getting better?"** Dr. Vermon Esplin was strong on this point and hoped all patients heed his warning.

> I think it goes back to the motivation is the key. Some people also in life have had things done for them. They have really not had too many challenges to overcome, and all of a sudden, this shows up, and it's catastrophic for them. Those kinds of patients, I have to spend a lot more time counseling what to expect and that this is

> not uncommon and that these are things that occur. So, you're right. What's going on in that mind is key. As surgeons, as therapists, as doctors, we do have a little bit of room to make an impression, but ultimately, what's going on in their head is the final say.
>
> Some of my patients are in there like zombies; they want you to take care of it; they don't want any responsibility for their outcomes. They just want you to fix the problem, and they don't understand their part in it. And the others, which we know, are very motivated and others, which, as we said, no matter what we do, they're not going to get better.

If I made a mistake in trying to manage my back pain, it was in not researching all of the options–including surgery. I finally saw the surgeon when it was clear that I had no other choice. I don't have any science to back up my belief, but I am convinced that the epidurals and other options I tried before seeing the surgeon made a bad situation worse. A surgeon would have explained, as Dr. Khurana did in the previous chapter, that my spine condition would likely not heal without a mechanical fix with surgery.

So, who should you be talking to and what should you be asking in order to create a surgical strategy that will work for you?

Some of the following is going to be doctor-speak. If there is something here you don't understand or something your doctor has not discussed with you, call your doctor and ask questions. By the way, you are not bothering your doctor when you call with questions. Quite the contrary, if you are not aware, there is a Patient's

Bill of Rights.[3] It is your duty to ask questions and be clear about what is being proposed and what proper care and service looks and sounds like. If you want the right outcomes, you have to ask the right questions and make the right decisions.

Dr. Christopher Hills leads off the advice with this discussion of general procedures. I asked him to give me some clarity on the variety of techniques and procedures that I had heard about. Dr. Hills walked me through it this way:

> In probably the simplest terms available in spine surgery we do two things. One is a decompression–taking pressure off the spinal cord, the nerve roots, or the spinal elements in some form or fashion. So, just creating more room for the spinal cord elements. On the other hand, there are times where we do fusions where you take away motion from a segment of the spine, one or multiple segments of the spine. There are some patients who are indicated for just decompression. There are some who are clearly indicated for fusion. There is some gray area in between those two.

We already learned a little about all the horror stories around fusions. I asked Dr. Hills to help prospective patients prepare to ask their doctor about this specific concern. Dr. Hills continued:

> Now, the main indications for a fusion are instability. That is, if you have a slippage of one bone on the other. Scoliosis is a form of instability. You have things such as fractures and tumors that can cause instability.

3. https://aapsonline.org/patient-bill-rights

> Those are clear indications for fusion. Part of the fusion is a decompression, whether it's what we call direct where you go in and manually open up the spinal canal, or the foramen, where the nerves exit out. The other method is indirect relying on the implants to do some of that work for you.

I mentioned that while I was searching for a surgeon, my anesthesiologist nephew asked to see my pre-op order. He was concerned about the word "laminectomy" in that order. Because of his concern I sought a second opinion. I asked Dr. Hills to talk about the importance of understanding your procedure and getting a second opinion.

Dr. Hills clarified:

> There are many ways to do a fusion, many ways to do a decompression. Nuvasive provides instrumentation to be able to do a minimally invasive fusion technique. It is just one of the ways to skin a cat when you're doing a fusion technique but, again, their methodology, their instrumentation, should not make a decision on whether you're doing a laminectomy or a fusion.

Dr. Justin Saliman also recommends a second opinion, but with some conditions.

> I think second opinions can be super-helpful and super-confusing. It totally depends on your scenario. If you knew that the doctor you were going to was good somehow, magically, which we don't, then you wouldn't need a second opinion. What I will say is that, especially in orthopaedics, if you talk to five orthopaedic

> surgeons, you will get five different versions of what to do. Some of them may say the same procedures, but they'll do it in different ways. Like very few are doing the exact same thing, and the reason is that there's not enough data, and the reason there's not enough data is that no one tracks outcomes. But, in the end, if we had enough data to truly dial in best practices, every single surgeon should do the exact same technique with the exact same technology or implants or disposables or whatever because we would know, we would have it dialed in, so we would know what works best. But because we don't have the data, we, orthopaedic surgeons, all do different things or different versions of similar things. There must be 15 different ways to do an ACL reconstruction or more. Same with joint replacements. It's very much up to that clinician and who knows what they've been exposed to or trained with, and they get very, very much set in their ways based on their experiences, and some of it may just be anecdotal experiences.

Dr. Khurana, encourages patients to ask a lot of questions. He asks a lot of questions of the patient as well. I came to him seeking a second opinion and asked should I be concerned about a laminectomy? I detail these facts to help you ask the right questions of your surgeons. This information was applicable to me and may help you to ask the right questions concerning your condition. It is not intended to help you make a decision for any specific procedure for your surgery. Dr. Khurana wanted me to understand exactly what was happening in my back. He explained:

> Because the spine is such a complex organ hosting, like we just talked about, a lot of nerves, it's right around a lot of visceral structures, and vascular structures, and the disc is kind of a highly innervated structure. In other words, there are a lot of nerve endings that go to the disc, and there's just many, many explanations as to why someone could have back pain or nerve pain. At a high level you look at where back pain and spine disability comes into the matrix as a population. I mean, it's an extraordinary part of the population where back pain leads to loss of work and loss of production. Maybe just second to the flu and the common cold. It's an extraordinary thing that we see, but as surgeons we realize that it's only a small subset of patients who really are ideal candidates for intervention. That's where the art of what we do comes in. I say the art—and the science. You have to identify where appropriate intervention is going to match patient symptoms and imaging.

He continued:

> From a patient standpoint it requires a few objective things, but some subjective things as well. **Number one, I think the most important thing from a patient standpoint, is to be motivated.** I think when decisions are made to do surgery it's really still is a team decision, even though it may be the surgeon's recommendation to move forward with the surgery, it does really require buy-in by the patient that they want to do this, that they

> want to get better. Being motivated and being positive is a very important part of the surgical process.

If I had it to do again (and I would do it again), I would be asking the doctor to explain how my imaging lines up with his or her exam.

- Do they correlate?
- I would ask, in all honesty, does the doctor believe you have the right mental attitude, the right commitment, to make enduring the rigor of surgery worthwhile?
- Does your doctor believe that you have a good chance of recovery? The surgeons are going to presume that they are going to do a perfect job.
- **The question you should ask your doctor is whether or not they feel you are going to do your part. And then, let your doctor be clear about what "your part" entails.**

Dr. Justin Saliman had some insight into this aspect of optimizing,

> So, the patient wants to feel like, what can they do? The doctor's going to do their part, and we're assuming that they're going to do a great job. What can the patient do to more fully recover or ensure the best outcome possible? There are a couple of things: Be compliant with the doctor's treatment plan, but then also do all the things that you're discussing in this book, which is, as far as I understand sort of diet, nutrition, mindfulness, attitude, meditation, being aware of what you're doing, and thoughtful in your decisions, both preoperatively and postoperatively, no question, no matter what the

> surgery, makes a difference. Even without surgery, it's been shown to make a difference.

Conditioning before surgery is the foundation of *The Optimized Patient* protocol. Your surgeon may have resources and relationships that you may benefit from. Your surgeon may not volunteer those services or even have the conversation with you unless you have comorbidity issues that would prevent the surgery. Surgeons do surgery and that is their focus. If you ask the right questions, they can and will do more for you than just put screws in your back.

If I do the surgery, what is it going to take to make a full pain-free recovery? What do I have to do, for how long, and how hard is it going to be?

That is a key question for your team *before* you decide to get the surgical fix. I hope you are starting to get the scope of what's involved in a successful surgery.

My interviews with the patients focused on, "If you knew then what you know now, what would you have done differently?" Although we all had excellent outcomes, we all felt that there were aspects of the experience that we might have done differently in hindsight. Linda B., our homemaker whose back pain started after her second child, talked about the importance of planning your time at home after the surgery:

> I tend to have a very great support unit. I had it set up before too. I have a group of friends, and I had 30-days' worth of meals made for me. I didn't cook for 30 days. I had people taking my kids to and from school. I had my mom, and I get choked up (Linda pauses to collect herself and her thoughts). If there's one lesson

> through this, it's I'm a doer. I'm a mom so I do a lot for my kids and it just comes naturally to me, but to receive that, and I'm sorry that I get choked up, but that help is priceless—to have that support is priceless. I think there's a lesson in going through this too. To learn to ask people for help, to get that support unit and to accept it and to be grateful for it.

More about caregiving and support in the Addendum contributed by Doug Amend.

Much of the literature on longevity talks extensively about the importance of family and community on a healthy lifestyle. I know people can't just conjure up family and community at the wave of a hand, but **you should reach out to make sure there is a support group around you.** I was a bachelor at the time of my first surgery, but I was lucky to have a group of dedicated friends and neighbors who provided much needed emotional support. I was able to take care of my personal needs, but the peace of mind that comes from having a support group close at hand is essential to making a successful recovery. I appreciate the fact that Linda B. mentioned meal prep. It was one of those areas that I wish I had known a lot more about *before* I went into surgery. I will cover nourishing your body for healing in depth in Chapter 11. (Since the publication of the first edition of this book, we created a delicious and easy to follow meal plan with recipes focused on healing.)

I thought it would be a brilliant idea to buy a ton of frozen dinners that I could just put in the microwave. I will talk later why that could be the worst idea ever.

You should ask your doctor how long you can **expect** to be homebound and unable to cook for yourself. As an extension of that, you should make arrangements for family members or friends or paid care providers to be close at hand in case you need assistance.

Joy H. was the most on target about this aspect of the surgical journey. Her neck pain was increasingly robbing her of her quality of life. It would make sense that she would be focused on asking questions of her surgeon. Joy was repeatedly told she should wait to have her surgery because of what "might" be her future. It is important to hear the strength with which she engaged her surgeons. She related:

> I would go into every new appointment with one firm resolution: that no matter whatever was told me, I'm the specialist on me. I would make that influence everything I told the doctor. "I respect what you're saying, I like your feedback, I like your ideas, but also hear me. I know my body. And maybe you think I shouldn't be in pain from this, but I am, so hear me on that." So, kind of holding my ground was something I had to learn—meshing the two: the surgeon's expertise with my expertise. And I do have some, on me. I was desperate to know what to expect, scared out of my mind, but I knew I had to do this. It felt like it was life or death, really. But I still would've liked to have known what to expect out of it all, and no one was there. You know that ream of papers they give you to sign, prior to surgery where you're dealing with all the possible outcomes and

> it kind of explains them—all the legal forms? You sign your life away, really truly.
>
> I think I asked prior to surgery, in those first few months, something like, "Am I going to have physical therapy, is that even somewhere in the plan there?" He said, "Well, initially life is physical therapy for you. You can barely move." I could barely brush my teeth, moving my arms for anything was really hard. I was so sore from the waist up. Sore, being an understatement of the year. I felt crushed from the waist up. Moving at all was therapy; it was work. He understood that, but I think he knew that going to a physical therapy gym appointment would just be impossible for me. He said, "Just keep moving and do your own therapy by just trying to do life."

Lucio D. was also very focused on what happens after surgery. He, too, had a lot of questions on "the horror stories" he had heard and was direct with his doctors. Lucio remembered:

> I swear I've had at least a good five people in my lifetime tell me, "Hey, man, once they cut into you, you'll never be the same." And that echoes in your head immediately. You go, "No way." This is a big physical change. And you start thinking about that, and you start asking your questions. My first question to the surgeon was, "Look, man, before the accident, I could go on an eight-mile hike, vigorously, and have no worries and be just fine. Can I still do that? Can I go put on my skis and go skiing if I get surgery? Will I ever be back to

> that?" And the guy paused for a long time. "Look, what you have going on in your neck is what I want to look at first. And we've done these before." And right away when he said to me, "Somebody else had this done and they went on to do some great stuff." He said, "You know, you're never going to be 25 years old again, but you definitely can still go on and do some great things with your body, if you want to. It's up to you." And he immediately told me Peyton Manning had the same injury. And he says, "Peyton Manning had the same injury as you; he had the surgery in your neck, just like that. And he went on to win the Super Bowl." So, right away, just those words made me go, "Okay, alright. So, this guy's like my age, maybe a little younger, and he got his ass handed to him. Now he's back in the Super Bowl. I can do another Super Bowl."

I wasn't interested in playing in the Super Bowl in my sixties, but I was very interested in recovering my gait. The limp I had developed was pronounced enough that is was starting to affect my knees and hips. In the early testing before I committed to Dr. Khurana, I had a doctor tap my knee a couple times with a rubber hammer. After a couple of increasingly energetic taps he looked up at me and asked, "How long have you been dead?" I tend to joke around with my doctors, and, frankly, I found it funny. It did identify, however, that there was real trouble in River City. Unfortunately, there wasn't a guidebook on what to ask and how to prepare. I don't believe anything I will detail in the rest of this chapter will change your outcome or help you cope with sarcastic physicians' assistants, but it may hasten your recovery and make the journey a little bit easier.

I have to confess that until I started writing this book, after two fusion surgeries and discectomy, I still had no idea exactly what a surgeon does. Understand, I know what they did as far as opening my back, putting in screws and instrumentation and closing me up again. I got that part. But, it was all the other things I thought a surgeon does that they absolutely do not do. As we have been learning there is a big and very significant difference between the surgical outcome and the clinical outcome. Your surgeon may be very active and engage with you on the surgical part. But, unless you ask the right questions and, more importantly, ask for the right referrals, your clinical outcome may really miss the mark.

So, what should you be asking your doctor before your surgery?

How limited will I be and for how long? What's the best way for me to manage?

You should have a frank discussion about how prehab may help your rehab. Ask your surgeon if based on your specific case, you would benefit from seeing a physical therapist before your surgery. Will it make the rehab process easier if you learn the exercises before you are hit by the surgical bus? With our eyes newly opened, let's listen to Physical Therapist, Solomon Joseph, once again. He brings it down to just walking in a swimming pool. But if you don't know to ask or if you just don't ask, you may miss an essential step that can speed up the best possible recovery. Here's how Solomon explained it:

> Well, every therapist should know, have some background in Aquatic Therapy coming out of school. They should. And if they don't practice it in the clinic, in today's age, go and Google the different things you can do. One of the things they need to express to their patients, talking to them, is how to help your core muscles while they're exercising in the pool. And exercises are not that difficult for rehabbing and prehabbing spinal injuries in a pool. Just moving around in the water is very beneficial. They can actually just get in the water and walk around for an hour and that would be very beneficial for the spine. If they're at that stage, just getting in the water and walking increases circulation around the spine in an unloaded system. So, they can get in there and have pain be their guide, as far as moving and jumping around and exercising and building strength while they're unloaded in the water system.

My personal experience with aqua therapy could not be better. In my particular case, I have so much nerve damage that I still cannot stand on my toes. I have calf atrophy that still causes gait issues. I have tried many land-based exercises, many of which have contributed to better function. That said, when I finally got into the pool and I was able to get up on my toes with the unloaded environment of the water, I was able to do exercises that were not within my ability on land. My physical therapists tell me that doing this is so important because it gives my brain and spinal cord a chance to reconnect with movements that ceased because of the trauma. Once the movement and the communication resumes, the healing begins. Without being in the pool it would have been impossible for me to start rebuilding my neural pathways.

Ask your doctor about wound healing. Much of what I have read would suggest that you may want to bring your sugar level down by cutting out sweets for a while before surgery. There is actual literature on this that goes by the acronym ERAS (Enhanced Recovery After Surgery). Read more about that in Chapter 9.

The following tip may see very odd, but I promise you it works. I had cut my hand pretty badly and happened to be at a Farmers Market when a honey vendor noticed the bandage. She explained to me that Manuka honey will help heal a wound. Being the skeptic that I am, I challenged her on the basis that she sells honey, so of course, it does everything! She explained that Manuka honey, when applied to a wound gives off a gas that has the same therapeutic action as hydrogen peroxide. While the honey is disinfecting the wound continuously it is also sealing and moisturizing it. To my shock and amazement, CVS actually makes a Manuka bandage! I used it on a recent knee surgery and it worked, so much so that my physical therapist said she had never seen anyone heal so quickly and with so little scarring.

Chapter 11 is all about nutrition. But, there is one particular thing you should ask your doctor before the surgery. It seems that after anesthesia, antibiotics and opioid painkillers, your gut goes to sleep. I mean, really asleep. It's a big deal when you pass gas after you wake up. A bowel movement in the first three days after surgery merits a call to CNN. It's a huge deal. In the hospital you will be given stool softeners as a strategy to get things moving. Ask your doctor about probiotics or products like Metamucil—prior to surgery—to help you with a rapid return to normal function. As we discussed earlier, the constipation that follows surgery is one of the most unpleasant and unsettling parts of the experience.

Dr. Christopher Hills has even developed a strategy to help patients bounce back as quickly as possible. Rather than put his thoughts in the "rehab chapter," I think they belong here as something you can share with your surgeon. Your doctor may or may not agree, but you should definitely ask. For clarity, this is the definition of the word catabolic from Dr. Hills, "Catabolic is a degradative process where you are calorie deficient, you are losing essential mass, if you will. It's just a degradative state that is definitely not what you want to go into starting a surgery." Dr. Hills expanded on that important definition:

> There's been a lot of research now that it used to be where no one would eat or drink after midnight, and they go throughout the night and show up for surgery the next day, and sometimes they're pushed into late in the afternoon for their surgery, and so they've gone 12, 16, or 20 hours without having anything to eat or drink, and they're already in a catabolic state before you start surgery. The studies have shown well now that, boy, that's not appropriate. We want to keep away from that catabolic state, because you're already in a catabolic state, and you give them anesthesia and these narcotics and everything—it just compounds the problem. And then you're chasing the tail the rest of the time postoperatively trying to get someone optimized, when we set them off on the wrong foot to begin with.

Dr. Hills continued with a caution:

> You should definitely review this with your doctor before you deviate from the instructions given to you by the doctor who is caring for you. We now implement it in our spine program where the patient will have an Ensure. There are certain types of liquid you can take even up to two hours before the surgery, and so we have patients who are getting oral intake two hours prior to surgery. We're feeding them sooner after surgery and trying to optimize their nutrition as opposed to putting them in a catabolic state even before the surgery begins. Again, there is a growing body of literature in Enhanced Recovery After Surgery that is changing the whole pendulum, or a pendulum shift, in how we're treating patients nutritionally pre- and post-surgery."

I know, that one is a shocker. It makes plain common sense to me. See if your doctor agrees. Now, close your eyes and relax, take a couple of deep breaths . . . the rehab process starts when you turn the page.

9

WIN OR LOSE IN REHAB

In order to understand how to navigate your rehabilitation, let's review where the surgeon's job begins and where it ends. There is a medical answer and a philosophical answer to this question. The medical answer flows from understanding the difference between the surgical and clinical aspects of back surgery. In that context, the surgeon's job ends when you are sewn-up in the operating room. How involved your surgeon is after that will be determined by how much surgically-related care is needed: like removing drains and monitoring your wound and vitals. Philosophically, patients believe surgeons are going to manage them from soup to nuts. That's a charming idea, but it is not how your recovery process works. More importantly, it's not how the recovery process should work. Rehabilitation is a highly specialized episode in the surgery and injury recovery story and is best left to professionals trained in rehab techniques and technology. The next three chapters cover activity, mindset, and nutrition. Each one of those areas is important enough, and complex enough, to warrant its own chapter;

however, they are all part of rehab. **Implementing what I share with you here is where your full recovery is either won or lost.**

The three surgeons who have shared their years of experience at the table are of a single mind about how much of achieving a pain-free outcome is on them and how much is on you. They all agreed on the importance of your commitment to do whatever is necessary during the rehab phase of the treatment. They also all agreed that as surgeons, rehab is not their area of expertise and they are reluctant to provide guidance in any aspect of your care that is not their core competency. That said, they were very definite on the ingredients for a good clinical outcome. Remember Dr. Hills was very pointedly clear about the tragic possibility of a surgical success ruined by a clinical failure. This chapter is about avoiding clinical failure after a surgical success. Simply said, **you can either build on the great work your surgeon did or ruin it with your lack of commitment.**

Activity is one of the keys to a winning recovery. Dr. Christopher Hills spoke about the need to get patients up on their feet as quickly as is safe after they awake from anesthesia. In my case, Dr. Khurana had me walking down the hall almost immediately after six hours of surgery! Here's what Dr. Hills had to say about movement:

> Early mobilization is critical. We've learned that, boy, you get a patient up within an hour of surgery and get them walking. The body has its own ability to cope with pain when someone's moving instead of lying in bed where they're focusing on their back pain, and lying on their back. You get them up and moving, the body helps

> stimulate itself and can help with pain. That's probably the biggest thing–that we're getting patients up sooner after surgery. I like to get my patients up within an hour of surgery and get them walking, and the goal is a mile a day. Obviously, in intervals to begin with, shorter walks, but trying to get a mile a day and ultimately building up to a mile at one time within the short postoperative period, regardless of what the surgery is.

Dr. Vermon Esplin shares an identical view as it relates to hand surgery.

> In reality, a lot of times, the body is your own best guide. For my carpal tunnels, I would say, "If it doesn't hurt, you can do it. If it hurts, then you need to give it more time and try it later." That's usually a pretty general guideline for people so that they can use things, but not abuse them as well. The literature is there that proves that if you have good oxygenation in a wound, you're going to be able to get it to heal barring any other unusual circumstance. As well, you're going to have fewer infections. You're going to have better tissue there when it does heal. You can take that to too far however; if you do too much, you'll inflame the area more and cause more scarring. But if you do surgery and don't move, scar locks down the tendons and in hand surgery, particularly, we're dealing with scar. If you get scar in a tendon or a joint, it severely complicates and compromises your hand function. So yes, motion is lotion, and we want you to get it moving as soon as possible

The importance of movement brings to mind the role of the physical therapist. It is important to note that physical therapy is not an automatic next step in the recovery process in spine surgery. In my particular case I had developed a very obvious limp. I have to admit, it took me several years to finally find a set of exercises that delivered results. A lot of finding what will work for you will involve trial and error and our good friend dumb luck. **The essential first step is to ask your surgeon if you should plan on rehab.**

Surgeons do not provide rehab services, but they do prescribe it. Just, remember, it is essential to ask. When I interviewed my Physical Therapist, Patti Sogaard, she shared a 30,000-foot view:

> The physical therapist can guide the patient to a proper balance for a better recovery. There is no magic pill, no magic bullet, there's just a magic formula: a good physician or surgeon, a therapist who appropriately helps with all aspects of recovery, and a patient who is compliant and participating. If any one out of the three areas are weak, then recovery is compromised.

What Patti means by "compliant and participating" is you have to get involved in the rehab process. I know it seems fairly obvious, but the biggest obstacle to spine patients fully recovering is not doing what they are told. Let's start at the beginning. If you have already had your surgery, you know I wasn't kidding about getting hit by a bus. Everything that didn't hurt before, hurts now and the things that hurt before the surgery don't hurt anymore. Here's the good news, if you are committed and participating, the things that hurt now will stop hurting soon. None of us could say that about our nerve pain. The pain that brought us to the surgeon's door was a pain that was never going to quit and was only getting worse. Surgical pain does subside over time and eventually disappears.

The effort to minimize damage during surgery with minimally invasive techniques helps to accelerate recovery. I have coined the phrase, optimized patient, to define a protocol on how to prepare for, survive, and recover from spine surgery. I think you will find it interesting to note that one of the most important aspects of the science around rehabilitation is coming from surgeons working with gastro-intestinal patients. Dr. Christopher Hills of Jackson, Wyoming, brought this emerging idea into the conversation. I think it is interesting to share here, not just for its details, but for the concept. Enhanced Recovery After Surgery (ERAS) means to accomplish exactly what it says. In layman's terms, it means to help you get better faster. Dr. Hills explained to me that this protocol would seem to have value for *any* major surgery.

I have included this information to alert you to the new thinking that is emerging about the best way to get better. Said another way, the optimized way to get better. There really is an enhanced way to navigate the surgical experience. As I mentioned earlier, all the patients felt one of the most challenging parts of their hospital stay was related to their G.I. tract: constipation. An ERAS-type strategy may help to accelerate G.I. recovery and help to rapidly return the gut microbiome to proper performance.

Doug Amend, our mountain climber, has this to say about it:

> In order to leave the hospital after the fourth day, they gave me the suppository and stuff, and I remember being able to go to the bathroom there. I need to go back and figure out whether it was the first week

> after the fall when I had the pain medicine that caused the constipation. Anyway, it was a good solid week without having the opportunity to evacuate and that was painful.

None of the patients had a frame of reference on how painful spine surgery would be. But, we all had a frame of reference on what a normal bowel movement is about and what life is like when your GI tract stops working! We then discussed if Doug had any awareness that the combination of anesthesia, antibiotics and opioid painkillers would bring his bowels to a screeching halt. He did not. I asked him if he had known how to optimize his bowels to minimize the constipation after surgery, would he have done something about it?

Doug laughed and said:

> If I would have understood that better before going into surgery, my wife's a big proponent of probiotics and things like that, she would have put together a regimen for me. "Hey, you're going in for surgery with anesthesia and opioids. So, let's have you eating this way before you go in." That would have been helpful, absolutely.

Doug went on to say,

> I can honestly say, no. I don't remember having a conscious connection of, hey, I ought to eat better because I'm gonna do surgery or I need to eat differently because I'm coming out of surgery. That's a missing link to successful recovery. My wife, again, is very attentive to nutrition, doesn't like my Mountain Dew habit, and as such, would have really delved into that as my caregiver

> to say, 'No, no, no. Here's what we're gonna eat. Here's what we're gonna do. This will make you better.' If we can improve the patient outcome with the nutritional aspect, I think that's definitely a void today.

Doug also had a very interesting conversation with Nathan "Rock" Quarry that shaped his recovery mindset. Nate is a retired American mixed martial arts fighter. Nate's comments about his spine surgery at the end of Doug's story are simply amazing, especially when you consider that the guy made his living brawling in a cage. Here is how Doug tells it:

> Then as I got about a month out, I was a little depressed because I'm in the back brace, confined to my home, on the first floor, can't go upstairs, can't go outside, through the Christmas season, because this is December 9th to January 9th. Doc says you can't go out of the house. You can't go off the first floor. You're using a walker. You've got to baby this thing. It's like all right. So, I buy into it, but, mentally, I'm struggling. I said, "Hey, can I talk to Nathan Quarry? I saw the video of him back in the MMA ring after he had XLIF surgery (a type of fusion) getting the crap beat out of him, thrown around the ring, and, in my mind, it's like, if he can do that and I'm having a similar surgery, then I should be able to do that. I want to talk to this guy and find out how he got back to that point."

Doug continued:

> Nathan lives in Lake Oswego, Oregon. He was, at the time, a ranked MMA fighter in the UFC. As such,

Nathan reached out to me and says, "Hey, I heard your story, before you even ask any questions, I've got to tell you, you are an absolute beast, because I didn't have to go through half the crap you did. So, I understand your surgery. I understand your story. You don't owe anybody anything. Do what you want to do. Just know, dude, I'm glad I'm not you." He goes, "How can I help you?" And I said, "I saw you got back in the ring. I'm feeling kind of puny. Help me get to where you are today." He goes, "Well, you're four weeks out of surgery. You've got another five months to go. You're not going to do anything." I go, "Nothing?" He goes, "Nothing. You're just gonna watch Netflix. I said, "I don't watch TV." He says, "You got a big problem, because trust me when I tell you, you're not gonna do anything. I don't care if you feel better; don't do it. I don't care if you think you can do it; don't do it. Six months you gotta tell me, right now you're not going to do anything." He said, "You do that, and you'll be successful."

Then he asked, "Have you ever broken your arm?" I said, "Yeah, I broke my wrist." Nate says, "How old were you?" I said, "Fourth, fifth grade." He says, "So, do you think about it today? Does it prevent you from throwing a ball, climbing a ladder, doing anything you want to do?" I said, "Well, no." Nathan asked, "Okay. Have you ever broken a leg?" I said, "Yeah, I broke my leg playing hockey." "Well, how old were you?" he asked. "About 26." He goes, "Do you think about it today?

> Does it keep you from playing hockey?" I said, "No, I don't think about it at all." He says, "You broke your back. It'll heal if you'll let it. You'll never think about it again. I'm telling you. Did you see me in the ring? I don't think about my back."

Personally, I was fully astonished by that story. I worried about the BLT (bending, lifting, and twisting) warnings from the doctors right after surgery. It's good to know that down the road you can bend, lift, and twist your opponents in a cage fight. That is, if you like that sort of thing. In case you are not clear about exactly what Nate is saying, it is this: rest is a critical part of your recovery. Your body will be working overtime to heal the incision(s) and process the bruising and inflammation that are the result of the surgical intervention. As I detail the comments in the next three chapters the mix of ingredients needed to recover will come into focus. They may seem at odds, like activity and rest. There is a delicate balance to be struck and a progression to be followed. I hope you are starting to feel the need for the kind of coaching provided by a highly trained physical therapist.

Dr. Hills also observed the importance of patient awareness, commitment, and involvement in the recovery process. I mentioned to him that I underline that it's a commitment on the part of the patient to get involved in his own recovery. Dr. Hills enthusiastically added:

> If a patient starts really tracking their outcomes, going back before what they were prior to surgery, and then monitoring it at surgical time, and then at periodic intervals thereafter, they will see their serial results, as

> they're marking their own outcomes on these surveys. We've learned it's not the surgeon doing those outcome measures, because we're biased. We have our own selection bias, because, boy, we think we do great work. It's really the patient-reported outcomes that are the ones to measure that are critical. The patient is undergoing the procedure, and they're the ones who are monitoring their success, or should be monitoring their success. I feel patient-reported outcome is the way to truly monitor the success of not only the surgeon but also the patient. And when they're actively engaged in monitoring their success they have more buy-in and are able to track their success and be able to adjust it appropriately.

This is a really crucial activity and is a long-established teaching in the success literature. One of my coaches in business, Blair Singer, teaches how important it is to "celebrate all wins and the wins of others."[4] While I was writing this book I actually called my trainers to tell them how extraordinarily well the success literature translated to surgical rehabilitation. When you think about it, focusing on what's working (wins) rather than focusing on what's not working (losses) will certainly have a positive effect on the outcome. Henry Ford famously said, "Whether you think you can or whether you think you can't, you're right!" Although his comment was made, I believe, to his engineers who were having trouble perfecting the V8 engine, it is relevant here. I believe you can easily

4. www.blairsinger.com

modify his observation to say, "Whether you think you can get better or whether you think you can't get better, you're right."

It has been proven in business and it would seem to be applicable to the rehabilitation process. Joy H. spoke directly to the mindset of focusing on the positive and celebrating all wins. Joy nearly gave up living because of her pain. What she experienced when she woke up and how she processed it may help you to prepare your own recovery and rehabilitation mindset and process. Joy shared:

> Honestly, all my worry hit after surgery. I wasn't terrified of surgery. Well, I mean I was terrified of being paralyzed or whatever, granted that didn't come to be. I obviously could still walk after surgery, and I didn't die, which is the other option. Yeah, a lot of those things didn't happen. Well, none of the three they gave me. They were like, "There's one of three outcomes here: the surgery will be a success, and you'll be fine, it'll solve your pain. Or you can die in surgery, or you can come through paralyzed." Those were the three outcomes that stuck with me, and I wasn't real happy that two-thirds of the options were pretty bad. Honestly, I didn't worry too much. I wasn't afraid of dying, and I knew I had my husband to back me if I came out paralyzed, and we'd had that difficult talk about how we'd go forward with life, if I was paralyzed from then on, at 28 years old. That wasn't the scary part. But afterwards I was feeling crushed. I thought, "Oh no, this was worse than I anticipated, I had no idea, did I just make the worst mistake of my life?"

> Somehow, I lived through it, and it got worse. I worried a lot, and I think that could have been alleviated if I'd had someone to talk with, someone who'd had an extensive spinal fusion. People said "Yeah, this is really hard. You have to give it time." Doctor Mendes did say when I was crying to him at my first month visit, I was sobbing in his office, I said, "What did you do? I can't believe I'm still hurting." He said, "Joy, it's not like you had your gallbladder removed. We did one of the worst things we can do to the human spine. Give it time." He looked me straight in the eye and said, "There's a biologic event of healing that has to take place, and it just takes time." It dawned on me in that moment, "Oh, he's right. It takes a long time for this stuff to heal!" Worrying after that point? I was just like, come what may; I think I need to settle in for the long haul. For starters, I probably wouldn't be alive, that's how bad it was. I told you already, I was really serious about killing myself. The fact that I'm still alive is a big deal. I don't have any pain daily anymore. It's 1,000% improved, yes. Everyone asks "Hey, how does it feel to be back to normal?" I kind of just look at them and think, "Well, I don't remember being normal. My pain started when I was 11."

It is so important to know how Joy turned the corner from trauma, fear, and what hurts to realize the positives of being alive and having the opportunity to heal. Our entrepreneur, Lucio

D., had a similar observation, but in a little different way. Lucio recalled:

> **Immediately after surgery, I think mentally you change, and you start prioritizing.** But I say, don't do that too much, because you'll start limiting yourself. I think it's very important that at least one or two people are there in your life who can let you know, hey, you're going to get better, you're going to be fine. You need those positive people. And those people should be identified way before you get to surgery. You should do that—that really is important for you to figure out those people who are going to at least tell you things in your ear that are good and positive for your outcome. Identify those people at first, because you're going to need to call on them and just have chats now and then. Let them know how you're doing.

I want to include a cautionary note about activity from Physical Therapist, Patti Sogaard. I think her view emphasizes that complex balance inherent in the rehab process: a little, but not too much; positive, but careful not to overdo. Here is how Patti put it:

> And you've seen these people in therapy, they have an injury on one body part, within a month or so, something else hurts cause they're not moving naturally, that's the physical side of it. On the mental side of it, which also is very important for the patient, people who don't know what to expect from the body while healing can be very not compliant and not heal well. They're scared, they're frustrated, they're impatient, and they

> need guidance for recovery through the whole process—to know what might be normal and what's expected of them to get the optimal outcome. Some patients with injury feel that if they have pain they should just stop moving and stop doing things because they have pain. Others feel that they should work through it and work harder and neither will lead to a quick recovery.

Somewhere in between thoroughly researched science and anecdotal personal experiences of the patients lies the wisdom of how to get the best possible outcome in rehab. For example, let's remember the "bee lady" at a booth in the Farmers Market selling honey. She was advocating the extraordinary healing properties of honey because it is true! The fact that I never heard of it didn't change the fact that many people were already using Manuka bandages they bought at their local pharmacy. I got mine at CVS. My Physical Therapist, Patti Sogaard, commented that she had never in all of her many years of practice seen an incision heal so fully and invisibly as the incisions I treated with Manuka honey. You should certainly check with your doctor about this. I will tell you I informed my doctors about it. My physical therapists are now recommending Manuka to all of their surgical patients for wound healing.

During the interview with Physical Therapist/Aqua Therapist, Solomon Joseph, I mentioned that the nerves to my calf muscles were so damaged that I could not stand on my toes on land. However, I was able to accomplish the motion of getting up on my toes when I was in water just above my waist. That seemed to be a critical piece of information and Solomon launched into why that was important in my recovery and how it may relate to your recovery. I shared with him that I was curious to see if I had any motor function and guessed that in the water might be a good place to find out. He said it was not only a good way to test function, it was the best way to recover function. Solomon said:

> Because you're 70 percent lighter in the pool, you're lifting a whole lot less weight in the pool. So, you can actually use those muscles in those specific exercises that you can't do outside the pool, which is very functional because you're actually on your feet and doing things versus just lying on a table and exercising and moving your foot up and down. You're actually giving yourself depth perception which is the body's way of figuring out space for balancing and everything else. So, when you're standing and doing these functional exercises in the pool, it translates a lot easier on land once you get stronger.

That was my exact experience. Once I was able to make the therapeutic movements in the low gravity environment of the water, I was able to copy it on land. I found that doing jumping jacks, and other exercises that were impossibly challenging on land were quite easy to do in the pool. The therapeutic benefit of actually making the proper movements in the pool seemed to allow the muscles and nerves to either re-learn or work around to restore function. It is important to note that the exercise in the water did not magically or instantly fix my problem. Quite the contrary, it took many months for me to regain enough function so that when I walked through an airport the porters didn't rush to offer me a wheelchair or an electric cart ride to the gate. I expressed my concern to Solomon that swimming was difficult during the rehab process. He was quick to point out the difference between swimming and movement in the water as part of a rehab regime. I asked him, for the sake of the readers who don't have time in the pool with him, what should they be discussing with their therapist if this approach is not the therapist's core competency?

Solomon laid it out this way:

> For rehabbing spinal injuries, you're in a vertical position, not a horizontal position, for exercise. I prefer to have your feet on the ground, touching the ground, for motion and balance. You can actually do it. If you have a problem with putting pressure on the ground with your feet, you can put a buoyancy belt around you to keep your feet off the ground and actually exercise that way. You're in a vertical position, not in a horizontal position, as in swimming.
>
> There's a whole new movement now for training, not just spine, but training lots of different injuries including elbows, shoulders, that kind of stuff. They actually get completely under water for training, getting into about 10 or 12 feet of water. Like if a baseball pitcher injures his shoulder, they actually get completely submerged with a breathing apparatus on the side of the pool and they actually throw their motions, in a slow motion, to help stabilize the muscles, because the muscles are too weak to go fast, at the speed that they need to move at to throw a ball. So that under water reduces

> the speed considerably, but they have the same motion, so the muscles work the same, the muscle memory applies but at a lot slower motion. And the muscles have time to react to the motion and the joints stabilize and do what they have to do underwater. And that is for boxers, for baseball players, for everything else—same kind of thing. Slow motion to help the muscles while the motion is happening at the joints."

Solomon also delineated what the optimal pool environment should be like at different phases of your recovery. My sessions with Solomon took place at a facility dedicated to rehabilitation for the disabled. The particular facility where I received my therapy was AbilityFirst.[5] I want to thank and applaud these folks who created this environment for the physically challenged. If you can't find a facility like this in your community, you might want to email AbilityFirst to see if they may provide a referral for you. Understanding that not every community may have facilities like AbilityFirst, I asked Solomon to detail some guidelines for you.

> If you're talking right after surgery, most gyms' pool temperatures are around 78 to 80 degrees, which is fairly cold for a lot of patients that would get in, if they had to get in to do exercises because they're not going to be exercising very strenuously—they're not going to be moving around very fast. They're moving around very slowly, so their core temperature is going to start to drop because the water is too cold and they will spasm. So,

---

5. https://www.abilityfirst.org/

> a rehab pool usually runs between 92 and 94 degrees. Once they get in the water, it's comfortable for them and actually helps relieve some of the pain because of the warmth of the water and, avoids spasms.
>
> There are facilities around that do have rehab pools that have the temperature around 92 to 94 degrees. They have facilities where they have Hoyer Lifts where you can actually get into the pool if you're in a wheelchair and you can't walk. They can actually put you in these Hoyer Lifts which will actually transport you from your wheelchair.

It is important to note that if the pool has one of those lifts, then it will likely have ready access to the pool with easy-to-navigate steps or ramps. I asked Solomon to address what to do if the only pool you have access to is your local health club. That pool is unlikely to be at 92 degrees. Here is what Solomon suggested:

> I tell patients, put on a rash guard and that helps to keep their body temperature from dropping. It's what surfers use when they're surfing during the summer time. It's a very thin Lycra, neoprene material. It's not thick heavy wetsuit material; it's a lot thinner so they can move around with it and it's a lot easier to put on and off versus a wetsuit. A rash guard goes all the way down to the wrist and it actually helps the skin stay warm a lot better, so you don't get any cold water going underneath the rash guard on your skin.

A final note from Robert G. that captures the rehab process in a nutshell:

> One piece of advice to give to people having surgery? Oh wow. In my own personal experience it is **just listening to your body after the surgery and pushing yourself, but not overextending yourself.** And, to me, that's been the most beneficial for me. Actually listening to my physical therapist more than my doctor because I dealt with the physical therapist a lot more.

The line between the surgical fix and the clinical rehabilitation could not be drawn more clearly. But, the physical therapists can only help those patients who have the will to get well and are ready to make the commitment to do whatever it takes.

10

THE WILL TO GET WELL

Let's take a deeper dive into "it's a commitment" and "mindset." If you are reading this book end to end, you know that education, prehab, rehab, and mindset are all part of the recipe for a full recovery. Knowing what needs to be done and getting it done are two very different things. I had two goals—to be out of pain and to be able to walk without a limp. Both of those goals seemed impossible to get. Between panhandlers at Starbucks and airport skycaps I was in a daily experience of being asked if I was all right or needed assistance. For a while, I felt pretty sorry for myself and then I met Noah Galloway[6]. Noah and I were both guests on the Home and Family Show on the *Hallmark Channel*. I was talking about financial matters, and Noah was talking about how he decided to live a full life even though he had lost an arm and a leg in military service. I knew how hard I struggled with pain and mobility challenges. I told him about my injuries and shared with him that I could not begin to imagine what he went though. In response, Noah, without even

---

6. noahgalloway.com/

trying, gave me a priceless mindset shift. He told me he had been depressed for many years after he was injured. It is part of what he talks about on speaking tours. Noah shared that he simply made a choice to stop feeling sorry for himself and start doing what he needed to do to get better. Noah knew that the journey to getting his life back had to begin with the will to get well.

Our mountain climber, Doug Amend, reminded me about one of the crucial elements of the rehab process that I have not yet touched on. When we think of rehab we picture physical therapists and exercise and the medical intervention that comes with the post-operative experience. The mind-body connection is especially critical in the first 30 days after surgery. Doug was anxious to share his thought on mindset. He said:

> Back to the let-the-body-heal conversation that we were having post-surgery, where if you shut down and allow the body to recover (obviously, nutrition is going to play a factor in that), one of the things that I was going to mention that Nathan (Quarry) pointed out was that I don't (and didn't) watch a lot of TV. I'm not into sitcoms or binge watching a whole series. That just isn't of any interest to me. So, the path that I chose was an opportunity to more or less reinvent myself from a personal growth standpoint. So, I started reading books on how to be better. How to be a better person. How to be a better parent, father, just how to improve my personal development: Darren Hardy, Elon Musk, Simon Sinek, Tony Robbins, all this stuff. I started going down that path of podcasts and Kindle books, so that's

> what helped me fill the time to allow the body to heal. In a roundabout way, I think that definitely helped my mental outlook 100%. I didn't at any point feel like the victim or feel that I got short changed. I felt really lucky.

Doug *is* really lucky and so are we for having him share his insight with us. There is definitely a balance between the activity that is essential to getting your body reactivated and the rest that is required to help you heal. Doug touches on nutrition and I will cover the role of food in healing in depth in Chapter 11.

If you are starting to realize that the healing process is complex with a lot of moving parts from swimming pools to bed rest to keeping your head on straight, you are on the right track.

Linda B., our mom who developed back issues after her second child, talked about the balance between activity and rest. It is interesting that almost all of the observations about the need for rest and a positive mental attitude came from the patients themselves. Linda recalled:

> One thing in particular . . . I really don't want to say I pushed myself, but I tried to find the balance between rest and walking. I would get up almost every, I think every two hours. I had a schedule in my brain and I would lie down for a while and then I would move for a while. And I'm lucky. I live near a park that has a circle, and I would go a little bit further each time and go as slow as I needed to go. It was something that I built up to and I got further and further and further, but I regularly did that throughout the day. I didn't play all day,

> but I allowed myself—there's a balance there—I allowed myself to rest, but I also participated in movement and I truly believed that helped me. I wanted to build and get stronger and better and I was a strong, active participant in my healing.

Yes, it's a commitment that needs to be backed up by the will to take action. I think Linda perfectly captures that spirit in her comment, "and **I was a strong, active participant in my healing.**" That is the mindset and activity connection that is the foundation of being an optimized patient. I had discussed with Dr. Branko the very good outcomes enjoyed by the folks who have contributed to this book. Along the way I shared with him the kind of accidental prehab they had done. He immediately brought in the mindset aspect as it related to healing. Dr. Branko said:

> The people who you're just mentioning, those guys who mountain climb and yoga, those are the guys who are gonna do good, regardless. The guys who we talked about earlier. They're the guys who have the positive mindset and the drive. Those guys, they're gonna make themselves better.

Those are amazing words from a surgeon, **"They're gonna make themselves better!"**

I hope you are getting the message: "getting better" is a lot different than "having surgery." Joy H., as we have discussed, struggled with back pain since she was a child. She has some very specific points of view about pain relievers that I will share with you later in this chapter. I had mentioned to her that during my rehab I had spent a significant amount of time walking on the beach. It was not only necessary exercise it was calming and life affirming. Joy reflected:

> Your comments about going down to the beach reminded me that was the one thing Tim did for me, after surgery. Because this strung out for months, right? I'm sure you've heard me. This is a months, months, months-long thing. One of the things that I really enjoyed was sitting out in the sun, 'cause I had my surgery in September, so it was winter as I was recovering, mostly. San Diego's winter, you can't argue with. He would take me down to La Jolla, the La Jolla cove, and we would park with a blanket, all kinds of pillows. If we were going to take a nap, we would do it there. We took our dog, and we'd just lay out with all these blankets and at least get some sun and some fresh air, and like you were saying, emotionally reset. It was powerful, getting out of the house and feeling somewhat normal, even though I didn't do anything. Tim had to carry all the stuff and then come back and get me with the car, but it was good, it was helpful to do those little exercises. If he hadn't done that for me, I couldn't have done it for myself, so it was pretty amazing . . . it's something to consider for patients who have a really hard recovery like that. To have someone come alongside who can get you out of the house, get you into the sun and the fresh air.

I believe Joy's comment dovetails into my chat with Noah Galloway. It's hard to be depressed and feeling sorry for yourself when you are out in the sun and fresh air. If it is at all possible, a support group of family or friends to encourage you and to provide some accountability was a critical factor in the recovery of all of our patients. Personally, I found it very easy to rationalize why I wasn't going to go walk the beach on any given day. It is hard to fathom that the thing that you dread is the doorway to your healing. It was very helpful to me to have someone either encourage me or join me on the walks.

Joy H. had some additional thoughts on the importance and difficulty of the will to get up and get the activity done. She lamented:

> I don't think I healed as quickly, because I couldn't move around, and the blood flow is what instigates the healing process. I wasn't walking as much as I wanted to, because I couldn't. It's a vicious cycle. I strongly advocate taking the medication to keep moving, and the moving is what will help you get off the medication. I just set goals for myself. I had plans to be off of it by six months out from surgery. My surgeon said a year, "It'll be a year for you to recover." But I set six months, 'cause I thought, well, maybe that's an optimistic goal.

There's a key word in the will to get well: optimistic.

Robert G., approaching retirement, made the commitment to put an end to his pain and take the surgical fix. As we have read, it was decades before he made the commitment. I don't know about you, but as you read his from-the-hip comments, see if you find your own thoughts in alignment with his fears and hopes for the recovery process.

Robert said:

> So, when I went into this I was thinking, "Oh man, I'm never going to be 100%." Maybe I waited too long or, you know, so many different things went through my mind. It's taken forever, as far as my muscle tone and everything, to get back up to where it should be. Initially, it's taken over a year for that, so it's taken a long time. Yeah, at least a year. I still don't think I'm 100% as far as what I was able to do before. And, it's been almost a year and a half.

What's really important about Robert's comments is what he says next. He is recovering over a long period of time. What's important? His will to get well. He does not let up! Robert continued:

> I've been bicycle riding, swimming. We had a pontoon boat, so I—it was a couple months after the surgery—just jumped in the water and just started slowly taking my time and just rehabbing myself that way. It felt great when I was able to swim because it stretched every muscle for me. I mean, it took a while to be able to go any type of distance. I think it was just not overdoing it, slowly knowing my body again, being able to go to a certain limit without overextending myself and just continual exercise and stretching.

As I have stressed earlier, rehab in the water is an excellent physical strategy and good for your state of mind as well. Robert further confirmed my position on what to correctly expect from a surgeon and what to correctly expect from therapists. In response to my question about who suggested and/or encouraged his commitment to activity and exercise, Robert went on to say:

> The doctor, I wouldn't say, so much, but the physical therapist. And, I did their physical therapy for about two months and then I just took everything and did everything at home and then added my own mix of stretching and exercise.

No discussion of the will to get well would be complete without looking at the pros and cons of painkillers. Opioids have taken a sound beating in the press recently. Concerns about opioid addiction were also prevalent when I was in my post-operative recovery. It's a double-edged sword. On one side, the painkillers allow you to move more comfortably. On the other side, diminished mental capacity, constipation and the risk of addiction are a constant concern. There really isn't a handbook or a formula for the use of painkillers. It seemed to me the opioid challenge is a place where your will is really challenged. Again, listen to the process of Joy H.:

> I didn't make the six-month goal. It ended up being nine months. But I had no one to help me with the wean. The pain specialist I went back to for the refills each month, she was flabbergasted when I told her that that final nine months was it. I said, "No, I don't need anymore, this is the final visit, you can sign me off here." She said, "How did you just do what you just did?" She recognized that no one had helped me to calculate how to back off of it—I did it without any help. It's pretty cool. She said, "You should come and work here and be an inspirational wean coach for all of our patients."

It is important to bear in mind that the pain medications, particularly the addictive opioids, have value to help facilitate movement. The more you safely move, the better the blood flow, the faster you will heal, the less you will need the drug. I will tell you that the painkillers do induce a desire to either kick back or just sleep. You really do have to have the will to get well and the certain belief that moving is going to help you heal. Doug Amend pointed out another positive aspect of the painkillers even though he has a tough-minded view about opioids. Doug said:

> Listen, you have to have the pain medicine so you can sleep and rest. Don't avoid taking the pain medicine to allow you to get the rest you need. If you're uncomfortable, take it. But there's no reason to live on it because when I started stretching it, from four hours to six to eight hours, my wife would say, "You don't look very comfortable," and I would say, "I'm fine," because I could feel it. I could feel the pain. Tony [his surgeon] is in one ear telling me don't deal with the pain, be comfortable and let your body heal, and my wife's saying, "Are you sure? You haven't taken a pill for seven hours. You can certainly take a pill." I'm like, "No, I want to go eight. I want to try to get the pharmaceuticals out of my body."

It is definitely a challenge to strike the balance between drugs, comfort and rest.

Another part of the will to be well is the commitment, to yourself, to do everything your doctors advise you to do, and then some. Managing your pain after surgery is the first test of will; the second is managing the pain management. I don't mean to be glib. Joy continued:

> **Commit. Say, "Yes, I don't want to be on these meds forever."** I only took them as long as I needed them, but I recognize that timeline is going to be dramatically different for each person. Perspective on what you had done was critical. I struggled with that a lot, because I was so competitive, as a person. I wanted to beat the odds and be this patient and spring back. I thought, "I'm super young, surely this should be easy," and my surgeon said, "A year recovery" and I was really disappointed at my one-month visit, when I wasn't fine.

Managing expectations is another point we have touched on earlier and it is useful to remember what the surgeons have said. Over promising to yourself and under delivering can be very undermining to your will. My wife constantly reminds me how much my gait has improved whenever I start to feel defeated that my gait is not yet where I want it to be. The will to get well can't be sustained in an environment of perceived defeat. As I said earlier, celebrate all wins. Even if that means celebrating that you were able to open your eyes this morning and transit to the bathroom without the use of a wheelchair, cane, or someone helping you.

Patti Sogaard sees a definite role for physical therapy in managing the recovery process and what painkillers have to do with the will to get well. Patti advised:

> Painkillers today are even different than they were twenty and thirty years ago. They're more potent and more addictive, and addiction is seriously on the rise.

> So, painkillers in the beginning can be very helpful. One, so that they can get joints moving, the first week or so it will help with decreasing the pain cycle, and it will help with physical therapy, but I think they should be weaned off and stopped as soon as possible because of the risk of addiction. With addiction, you also won't have the same recovery, 'cause all of a sudden, their mind is going in a different direction and no longer with recovery, potentially.

Her warning is clear: opioids have the capacity to relieve temporary surgical pain, only to inadvertently create long-term addiction. It is important to come with the mindset that painkillers have a short-term role in your recovery, but that proper rest and focused activity bring long term-healing and true pain relief.

Having worked with hundreds of patients, this is how Patti explains the proper use of painkillers:

> So, I feel they can be very important at the beginning, but it is better to wean people off as soon as possible and use other things to help decrease pain for recovery. Ice is one of them, eventually switching over to something that's a non-opioid medication or anti-inflammatory—anything to decrease pain that is not habit forming. **The healing process needs to be guided for that perfect outcome**, and it's the physical therapist who's going to be able to educate the patient on how to stay healthy, what to do, what not to do, what to look for, what's a healthy pain, what's not a healthy pain, so the patient can continue to move forward, staying

> positive. The mental aspect of recovery is as important as anything else, and knowing what the path might be helps too—knowing the ups and down of recovery.

Lucio D., you may recall, was foremost concerned about being able to look up at the sky after he was smashed from behind in a car accident. Already a physically active person he developed a very positive mindset about what would lie ahead for him. I asked him what he thought his role was in recovering from his injuries. Lucio said:

> I realize it does come down to me. And that's the big part of it that I think was right away clear from my doctor—I can do all of this, and if you follow what I ask you to do and do your part, this will be very successful. And, you know, some of these guys have done their math and have seen that people that do this, seem to do better than the ones that don't. And they showed me percentages, they said, "If you're not doing this, 12% of the people who didn't do this, actually failed." And that's where I went, wow, they got this down to a number.

My conversation with Lucio was around the idea that this book would become a guidebook or a handbook for people who are considering spine surgery. We were talking about a way to optimize in preparation and in recovery. Lucio immediately picked up on it:

> But I noticed there wasn't a system set up. It was a lot of the doctor having to do this. And, like I said, not only does it come down to you physically preparing yourself, I think a lot of it has to do with mentally being ready or being strong and having that will. It's huge, it's 50%

> of it. I think the whole thing for me to fight back and all the bad things that were happening in my life made me want to want it more and want to fix it more. And you really have to have that drive. I think that's huge. I think sometimes it's one of the things these people are missing who get into these accidents and this happens to them—they sometimes need that and they don't have it. They don't have someone that's going, "No, no, no. You're tough, you're strong, you can do it. You're a human being; we are unbelievable in what we can do."

How's that for a strong mindset? **"You're a human being; we are unbelievable in what we can do."**

I am going to make a little bit of a departure here and detail the importance of mindset from my personal perspective. All of the patients had fears, but they also had a hope to be pain-free and to be able to once again do many of the things that made life worth living. When you drill right down into it, we come back to the core idea that a successful surgery begins with the commitment to yourself to get better. A positive mindset is the first essential piece. But, as we are discovering, commitment to actually doing the work to get better is the other half of the equation.

The will to get well cannot be separated from the activity needed to actually get the body moving and the blood flowing to facilitate healing. Dr. Branko summed it up best. It was a little surprising to me that a surgeon was so focused on patient mindset. Dr. Branko offers a concise summary of the complex issues surrounding commitment:

But what it comes down to for me is you can pretty much tell right off the bat if the guy or the lady is going to do well or not. How? There's a lot of psychosocial stuff that's involved here. Some of these patients who are hung up with chronic back problems and who end up coming to your door because nothing's worked for them—they're in so much pain and they're depressed and nothing's working out—if you really look at those patients and you look at what's going on in their life, there is a lot more trouble somewhere out there—a lot more trouble. And much of this stuff ends up expressing itself in some somatic problem. In this case it may be that, yes, they do have some sort of problem with their spine and they never really took care it because they were never really motivated to do so because maybe they were depressed because of the condition they were in and everything else that's going on. Maybe they can't afford their mortgages. Maybe they have a problem with their loved ones. Maybe their whole life is upside-down. Or maybe they just can't cope with the challenges.

The patients who do well are those who are motivated, who have things going for them. The other big thing in today's society is . . . where is the family? Everybody's divorced, everybody's got kids who are moving around with different family members. There's a lot of social problems that are involved here. The patients who do well are those who have a good family core, they have a good group of friends around them, they have a

> good job, they're motivated, they're looking forward to doing things in their life. Those are the patients who do well. No matter how bad the condition is, you do something for them, they're gonna make sure they get better. They're gonna stay on top of the physical therapy. They're gonna go beyond what's asked of them and they do well, versus the guy on the other side of the spectrum. He had his surgery and then he's just sitting there, he's pitying himself. Maybe he'll get better, maybe he won't, maybe he doesn't wanna get better, after all.

Those are very tough words from a doctor. They are his observations over a long period of time about patients who have done well and those who have done poorly. In Chapter 5, "The Surgeon's Perspective," we started to hear from the surgeons about their assessment of mindset as part of their overall assessment of a patient's viability for surgery. You might think that how the images correlate with their exam, patient weight, general health, smoker, etc., would be the criteria. But the surgeon's observation of the patient's mindset, their willingness to do the hard work of getting better, was also an essential factor in the surgeon's decision to offer the patient a surgical fix.

Dr. Saliman has observed similar patterns in patient behavior that has either led to a poor or an excellent recovery,

> Getting yourself in a good mental state to be able to tackle this recovery has been shown to improve your outcome, aside from everything else. And so, I would like you to read this book," or, "I would like you to enter this program. And in the end, that is the most

> compelling thing I think to say to a patient, is to actually give them a little gentle, very simple data around, "You can do it this way or you can do it that way," meaning, you can do these things ahead of time and afterward that are good for your health, and it will improve your outcome, or you cannot do them, and you may get a worse outcome, and here's how much worse.

I keep circling back to linking a positive mindset to actual activity. As I have been working on correcting my gait for over a year, I want to repeat that accountability is another essential ingredient to achieving your goal of a full recovery.

A physical therapist is a fantastic way to make sure you are doing correctly what you need to do and also doing it as often as it should be done.

It is hard to avoid doing the work necessary for your full recovery when your therapist is standing right in front of you! As committed as I am to getting well, the only time I absolutely do my gait training is when Patti or Solomon or Russ or any of the therapists who are guiding me, are literally doing the counts and making sure I am doing them all and doing them correctly.

When I began to formulate what the characteristics of an optimized patient might be, I really hadn't considered mindset. My personal focus was on the physical aspects, especially core strengthening in prehab. I thought if I could get that done correctly, I would be able to coast through rehab. I could not have been more shortsighted. Carefully programmed activity is key to the best possible outcome. What I hope you realized along with me is that mindset has a lot to do with your will to get well whenever pain is involved. Increasingly, over time, it became very tempting to say, "I hurt," "I can't," "tomorrow"—anything to allow myself the excuse to stay down and "let my body do the healing." I was quickly corrected by my physical therapist. A very rapid mindset shift was required to get me on the road to complete healing. "I hurt so I am going to take it easy" became "I hurt, but I am going to do the activity and I don't care if it hurts right now because this is what I have to do to get well and stay well." "I can't" became "I can and I will if it's the last thing I ever do because I want my life back." Most importantly, "tomorrow" became "I will do this today, right here, right now, if I do nothing else because nobody can do this for me."

Those are very significant mindset changes that can be the difference between a successful spine surgery and failed one. Dr. Hills clearly warned about the real possibility of having an absolutely flawless surgery and then succumbing to a total clinical failure because the patient did not commit to doing the very hard work of healing. As we have learned, the body is programmed to heal. Most of the healing work is done by your body without your prompting. You don't need to think about your heart beating, it just does it. Just like your heart, you don't make your body heal; it will just do it automatically. That said, we do have to think about how to keep our hearts in good working order. Likewise, we need to think about how to keep our ability to heal in good working order. This is, again, part of the mindset and the will to get well. Are you giving your body what it needs to heal? Are you thinking about what you are putting into your mouth? Is what you are eating part of the solution or part of the problem? One of the most important activities in the healing process is eating. What you are eating is just as important as how much time you spend in the pool, how much sleep you are getting, or how positive you are about your chances for a full recovery. The commitment you make to eating foods that will help you heal is the subject of our next chapter. The majority of the information in Chapter 11, "Fire Up The Recovery Engine!" will be provided by a professor of nutrition at my alma mater, Syracuse University. Proper nutrition, and your willingness to expend the effort to achieve it, is another aspect of the will to get well. It is so important that it begged for its own chapter.

11

FIRE UP THE RECOVERY ENGINE!

Does it make sense to you that fresh fruits and vegetables are better for you than frozen dinners and fast food? Do you need a scientific double-blind study to prove it? If the answers are yes to the first question and no to the second, then this chapter will make a lot of sense to you. Many of us in the post-operative scenario default to frozen dinners and fast food because it's either easier to do or the only thing we are capable of doing. Once ambulatory again, fast food takes center stage because it's easy and provides some degree of comfort. Here's the thing—both of those inclinations, frozen and fast, are the worst possible choices to support rapid and full healing. It never occurred to me to look for a book on what to eat after surgery. If it had occurred to me I would have found absolutely nothing. (I will provide recipe resources for relevant sites that have a vision that is congruent with *The Optimized Patient* strategy.) I am thinking about a cookbook to provide recipes and a protocol for healing. This book doesn't have any recipes, but it will help you to understand how to think about food that heals and in so doing help you to fire up the recovery engine.

Pritikin, Paleo, South Beach, Keto—the parade of diets is endless. Interestingly, they have the common thread of purporting to provide a health benefit in addition to weight loss. Lower your sugar or your cholesterol, increase your energy, burn fat, and improve cardiac function. **I found out *after* surgery that what you eat, or don't eat, can play a critical role in injury recovery.** This is another piece of the "dumb luck" that informs several aspects of this book. I was fortunate to have had informal coaching from a health sciences acquaintance who had some very definite ideas about healthy and *healing* eating. What he said made common sense to me and seemed to be quite effective. For the purpose of this book I reached out to a PhD in nutrition to make sure I was on solid ground on what I will report here. That said, much of what I will share is hard science or has been scrutinized in rigorous clinical trials. What we would all agree is known is that your body needs to be nourished for it to heal. I will suggest that what you need is not in a bottle or a box—it's in the fresh food aisle of your grocery store! I hope this anecdotal chapter on nutrition as a healing strategy will make common sense to you and that you will join me in firing up your recovery engine!

The funny part is that you intuitively know what I am going to share with you here is true. I am betting you've known it since you were in grade school. Do you remember learning about the trade routes to the New World? To me some of the most interesting details were the stories about the English sailors who got sick on the long voyages across the Atlantic Ocean. I was fascinated by the fact that they got sick from what they weren't eating. In 1747, Dr. James Lind guessed that something was missing from the diet of all the sailors. He gave each of the sick sailors different treatments and observed and carefully recorded their progress—or lack of progress. He divided the sailors into six groups of two sailors each. He had no clue about what was causing the ailments, but he did believe it was something that was missing from their menu.

Do you remember what it was?

Dr. Lind had the first group of sailors drink one quart of cider daily. The second group gargled with sulfuric acid (and wished they were in the first group). The third group was given two spoonsful of vinegar, three times a day (now apple cider vinegar is a popular home remedy). The fourth group drank one half pint of seawater daily. The fifth group drank barley water. The sixth group ate two oranges and one lemon daily.

I know it may be hard to believe, but all of the sailors in every group felt worse, except for one group. No, it wasn't the group drinking seawater. I am sure you have guessed by now it was the group who ate the oranges and lemon. By the way, it only took the sailors in that group less than a week to fully recover and return to their normal duties. By trial and error and observation, Dr. Lind had discovered that scurvy was curable by giving the ill sailors oranges and the lemons.

Scurvy is a disease caused by a vitamin C deficiency. So, when the sailors began long voyages where it was difficult to keep fresh fruits and vegetable, they ate large quantities before setting sail. Vitamin C is found in fruits such as oranges, grapefruit, lemons, strawberries, and melons and in many vegetables such as broccoli and bell peppers. But, the sailors of that day believed that it was the acid content that cured scurvy. Doctors agreed, and thought that lime juice would work best because is more acidic than lemon juice. Limes were, therefore, consumed in great quantities just before departure.

As a result, the English Royal Navy sailors became known as Limeys!

Scurvy wasn't a disease at all; it was malnutrition. So, what does this have to do with preparing for and recovering from surgery or a major injury? Foods can and do heal. It's rather interesting to take a look at so many ailments that have been remedied with food.

From ancient days Hippocrates said, "Let food be thy medicine and medicine be thy food."

There is an increasingly serious focus on nutrition and how it helps—or hinders—your body's ability to recover from disease and injury. When you understand how important nutrition is to optimizing your body's ability to heal, you will understand how extremely important nutrition is when addressing trauma and surgery.

Can people eat their way to better health? The better statement would be that people can and do eat their way into illness resulting in high cholesterol, diabetes, high blood pressure, and a dozen different digestive diseases. During my interviews with the patients, this is the one area where they wished they had been better informed. Looking back on their prehab and rehab experience, they regretted not knowing more about how good nutrition could have helped them recover faster. If you think that nutrition isn't important, think about this: every patient sitting at the table said the worst part of their surgery was the constipation they endured for days after surgery. Constipation, worse than spine surgery?! Yes. The effect of anesthesia, antibiotics, and opioids on your gastrointestinal tract is dramatic, as we have learned. So dramatic, that constipation is top of mind for each of the patients interviewed for this book. The nutrients you need to fire up the recovery engine that is your gastrointestinal tract are going to be very hard to access when your engine is stalled and your bowels aren't moving. Our experts are going to tell you why that happens and how to get things going again.

Before we explore a nutritional strategy, it's important to hear the experiences of our patients and the observations of our doctors. Let's recall on this imaginary evening we have all gathered at the dinner table to talk to you about your upcoming surgery. It wouldn't be right to overlook the role of good food. To that end we are also going to hear from Dr. Kay Bruening, who is a PhD in nutrition at Syracuse University in upstate New York. Nutrition is a relatively new and emerging science. I would need a complete and separate book to properly cover the subject. This chapter will contain a number of resources and reference for you to explore on your own. All I can say to encourage you to do the homework is that I was able to stop taking four prescription medications when I started minding seriously what I ate. Oh, if you need more incentive, I lost—and was able to keep off—over 20 pounds, which was 11% of my body weight.

Please forgive the long introduction, but this is one area where commitment is really put to the test and is most important. Altering my eating habits to optimize healing was a huge challenge. No meat. What? No wheat? Huh? No . . . wait a second! Let's change the conversation because a diet is different than a nutrition plan to nourish your body for healing. Let's turn our attention away from what we can't eat to what we should eat to benefit our body's natural healing process. Like me, once my screenwriter friend Adam committed to eating a diet that was mainly fresh vegetables and fresh fruit, he also lost over 15% of his body weight. After a couple of months of enjoying his weight loss and improved health, he never went back to eating as much meat and wheat. Neither did I.

When I questioned the patients and doctors about the role of nutrition, they either wished they had been in this conversation *before* surgery or said they were just becoming aware of the foundational role of fresh (and organic) food in the recovery process. Another one of my pure dumb luck meetings occurred at a Syracuse University alumni gathering. I received a graduate degree from Syracuse University and frequently attend their alumni events in Los Angeles. Syracuse is very active in Los Angeles primarily for its Newhouse School students who are studying broadcast and social media. At one of the alumni gatherings, I met Dr. Kay Bruening PhD, RDN, FAND, who is an Associate Professor in Nutrition Science & Dietetic Nutrition. . She received her PhD in Clinical Nutrition from New York University. At the end of the formal presentation, I told her about my thoughts on nutrition as it relates to post-operative spine surgery patients. I asked her everything from why does the food pyramid change every couple of years to what is the latest science on food and trauma. Not only did she clear up the food pyramid confusion but she also had a better resource that turned out to be the perfect place to begin to understand how food helps your body to heal.

Dr. Bruening started by updating me that it was no longer a pyramid, it is now a plate. She said:

> The food guide pyramid went away sometime during the Obama administration and was replaced with this plate. I don't know if you remember the pyramid that had like the colored stripes on it going up and down? That pyramid was hard for people to understand. So, they moved to MyPlate, because studies had shown it was easier for people to understand. But I'm not the expert on this, Marion Nestle is.[7] When the United States government, particularly the cabinet, comes out with recommendations, those recommendations are somewhat based on the science and also somewhat based on the influence of special interest groups.

Really? So, who can we trust and turn to for what healthy eating even looks like? Dr. Bruening continued:

> So the Harvard Healthy Eating Plate[8] is based on large scientific studies conducted by the Harvard T.H. Chan School of Public Health Department, which has been led by Dr. Walter Willett for decades.

---

7. https://www.foodpolitics.com/

8. https://www.hsph.harvard.edu/nutritionsource/healthy-eating-plate/

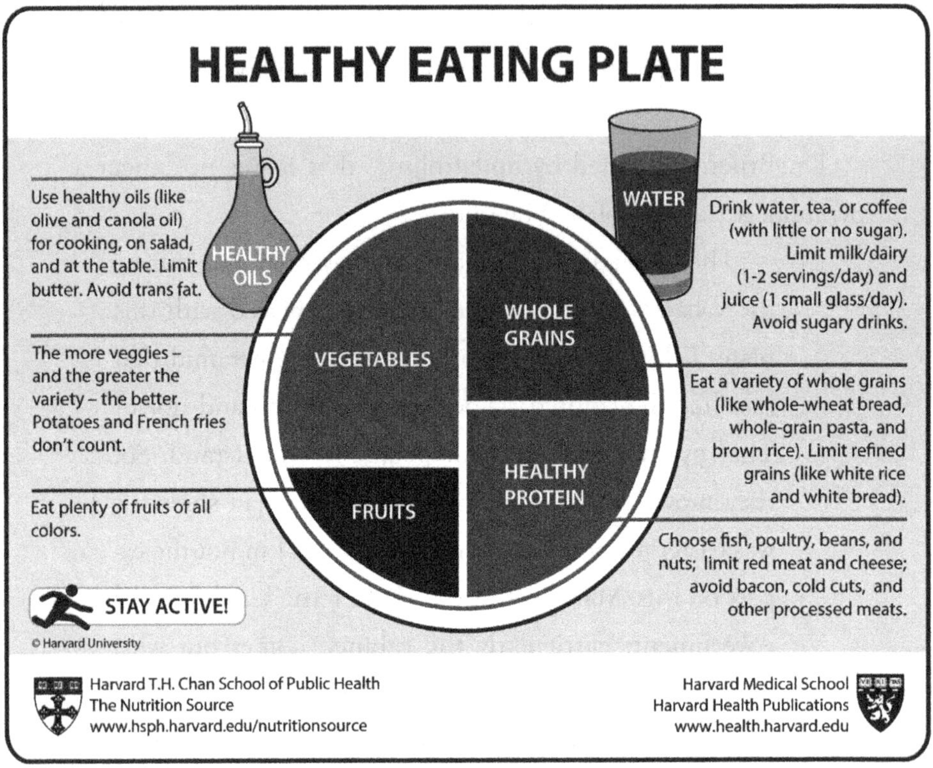

Hmmm. I don't see McDonalds or frozen dinners on the Harvard plate anywhere. I share this with you because the theme of this chapter is to fire up your recovery engine. The "fire" is in the nutrients found in the fresh fruits and vegetables in your grocery store. As a side note, I gave up the animal protein part of the Harvard food plate for about a year. I wasn't vegan, but I tried to adhere to a vegetarian eating plan with an occasional fatty fish, so I wouldn't go out of my mind. After a while, I no longer missed the meat. Oh, did I mention that I lost 20 pounds without trying or even thinking

> about it? Yes, I did. You cannot imagine my joy and the benefit of losing that weight as I improved my nutrition. There is a scientific reason for that I will share later in this chapter. Make a note of this word: *microbiome.*

We already talked about the wound healing magic of Manuka honey. Along that line, I asked Dr. Bruening if there was an eating strategy for healing that was as surprisingly effective on our inside as Manuka honey is on our outside. Dr. Bruening said:

> There's a new advanced medical nutrition therapy textbook out, and it has a chapter on wound healing. It talks about the three phases of wound healing and some of the specific cells and specific chemicals that those cells make that facilitate healing and reproducing all those cells and letting them do their job of making the little chemicals that help promote healing. It takes nutrients. Nutrients are required for all of that. So, it's an interesting chapter. It's kind of technical and kind of biochemical, but it does provide the scientific basis for it.

I said at the beginning of this chapter that I don't have scientific data on how nutrition affects healing spine surgery. However, there is significant information out there for you to draw your own conclusion and to form your own strategy. One thing I can say, and Dr. Bruening said it too, "It's a wonderful time to improve their dietary intake in preparation for this major surgery."

If you just said to yourself, "How do I do that?" It was the same thought I had and the same question I asked Dr. Bruening, "what diet does that?" She answered:

The Mediterranean diet does. It's published by Oldways Preservation Trust. They have a website[9] and they've produced materials. So, that would be a great place to start. I think it's easier for people to learn from something that's a graphic and makes a picture in their mind than it is to read a lot of words. But the Mediterranean Diet pyramid that Oldways puts out, at its foundation, has physical activity and enjoying meals with other people. Then at the huge bottom, probably a third of this pyramid is fruits, vegetables, grains, mostly whole grains, olive oil, beans, nuts, legumes and seeds, herbs and spices. Then there's a thinner slice of this pyramid above that includes fish and seafood, and an even smaller section above that one that includes poultry, eggs, cheese and yogurt, and the teeny tiny little triangle at the top mentions meats and sweets. Then outside the pyramid is a photo of red wine in moderation and drinking plenty of water.

Dr. Bruening continued:

So, that's the Mediterranean diet. And all the fruits, the vegetables, the whole grains, the legumes, the nuts, the seeds, those are the foods that contain many of those phytochemicals that I sent you the folder about from the American Institute for Cancer Research. They're not essential nutrients. You can grow a human without them. But those compounds provide additional health

9. https://oldwayspt.org/

> benefits. So, I would think they may be very important in healing, and they're also very important in the area of cancer prevention and recovery. That's why the American Institute for Cancer Research has invested so much in this research and in creating educational materials for the public. So, and as you have said yourself, surgery is a physiologically stressful procedure, and many chronic illnesses are also physiologically stressful and they change your metabolism and your biochemistry, and the way out of that requires nutrients, and I would say probably phytochemicals also.

Dr. Bruening summarized saying:

> So I would continue to get *at least* five servings of fruits and vegetables a day, preferably more. I would make as many of my grain choices as possible whole grain. I would make sure I was eating some dried beans, peas, or legumes every other day or so, and on an off day, I would probably have a handful of nuts. I would keep myself hydrated. I would make sure I ate some high quality protein, fish, chicken, eggs, etc. All high-quality protein.

As I mentioned earlier, I stuck with fish.

We spoke briefly about the "Blue Zones"[10] detailed in the book by Daniel Buettner because they are famously known for diets that support healthy living and super longevity. Dr. Bruening underlined:

---

10. https://www.bluezones.com/books/

> Blue Zones are places on the planet where people live traditionally and they have the longest life expectancy. There are several of them. The people there, in addition to eating mostly fresh, local, whole, minimally processed foods, are also doing some other things that play into this, like socialization and sharing meals with people and having a culture that promotes that—and possibly some other things like physical activity and emphasizing faith and that sort of thing.

Remember, this is commentary from a nutritionist! Those last few items relate back to the previous chapter about mindset or, said in this context, state of mind. It was not surprising that none of the patients knew much about nutrition as part their rehab plan. I brought up the subject of nutrition and microbiome at the imaginary table and this is what I learned.

It was interesting to me that our homemaker, Linda B., had a part of the puzzle. You may recall what Linda said:

> I walked every day. I have a lot of hills around my house. I visualized building my heart stronger for the surgery. I pushed myself to continue walking because I wanted to be stronger for the surgery. I gave up drinking too. I'm not a big drinker. I like wine, but I didn't drink for about a two year period, I'd say maybe six months before the surgery and then like after because I felt I wanted to do everything that I could to make my bones feel better. So, I ate more greens, anything I thought would help my body mend faster. This surgery was gonna put me back quite a bit and I needed to do

> everything on my part and in my power to participate in making my healing better. So yeah, if there was something that I could do and if it was as simple as not having a glass of wine or eating more vegetables or going for that walk, I definitely did it.

Take a minute to closely look at the Harvard MyPlate. Remember what Linda said? She had it exactly right! She doesn't have a science degree, she has the common sense to listen to her body and do what comes naturally. **Stay active!**

After his car accident and surgery, Lucio D. also considered how food figured into his recovery. It is interesting to note that only Lucio mentions his doctor in the food equation. Again, surgeons do repairs, nutritionists guide your food choices. Lucio said:

> We did speak about what my nutrition should look like from here on out. I think only pertaining to the post-operative experience. And then what you just said, I think that was really what the conversation was about was—now that you're healing, try and eat this stuff. The conversation did not go into "from here on out you should probably more stick to this stuff because it helps your bones or something," you know what I mean? We didn't have that conversation. We just had the, "try and stay on this diet while you heal, and it's going to take you the next year to fully heal." So, try to spend the next year eating like this and getting your exercise. And we spoke about stretching and all that stuff. But I think nutrition was not that big a part of that conversation.

Like me, Doug Amend had the dumb luck of having some focus on his diet before he fell off the mountain. Doug recalled:

> Strangely enough, I had entered a nutritional program called Real Appeal. It was a weekly coaching via video conference–meal plan, exercise regimen, an app on your phone to track everything. I had entered that program in June, prior to my fall, so ironically I started that in June at 198 pounds, and then by August I was 173 pounds. I'd cut 25 pounds off, and then in September I fall off the mountain. Fortunately, for me, I was definitely in an improved health/physical/mental state just as sheer luck would have it. Had I done that same fall the year prior when I was 25 pounds heavier and not paying attention to my nutrition, there's a good chance the recovery would have taken longer. But, I just happened to have used a three or four month program prior to surgery to improve my health, cardio, all this other stuff, and yes, I can absolutely attest that I believe I healed better because of it.

The doctors, although not specifically advocating an approach to any specific nutrition plan, certainly confirm the importance of good nutrition in recovery process. Dr. Khurana added his support saying, "Anything about nutrition, and the biome, and things that are kind of optimizing patients' outcomes, I am just extraordinarily interested in. I'm a subscriber. For me it's just about learning about it."

If you have not been reading about the biome and don't know what this is about, not to worry, it's covered later in this chapter.

I asked him if I was right-minded in talking about firing up the recovery engine with fresh food? Dr. Khurana offered:

> Yes, exactly. I think the comment about the GI tract shut down post-op after opiates is pretty widespread. There's variation between patients in terms of how bad their GI shutdown will be, but there are a number of new generation drugs that block the opiate receptor in the gut . . . and a number of others that should prevent the gut from shutting down. So those will be good things that actually keep the gut moving. But, I do agree that if you don't have the proper nutrition, both pre- and post-operatively that can really modulate the outcome and that's something important to pay attention to.

3,000 miles away and in a completely separate conversation, Dr. Branko picked up the ball as if he was sitting across the table from us. The doctor said:

> This, what you're just talking about, opens a whole 'nother can of worms. And when you come to talk about nutrition, we have so much evidence in our field that diabetes, high glucose levels, destroy discs. All this stuff that's in food, the preservatives, God knows what else is in there, is bad for discs, is bad for the body. A lot of the people out there, the everyday Joes, they cannot afford to eat well. They're eating all this processed food that, bottom line, is very bad for you, and they're putting that stuff into their bodies before surgeries, they're putting that stuff into their bodies after surgery. What percentage of their problem was caused by this in

the first place? We don't know, but it isn't helping the situation.

Dr. Justin Saliman added,

> "Before you have the surgery, your body is static a lot of the time because you're hurting and because you have this pathology. So, you're not moving around as much or as well. And then, you have anesthesia, and you're laying very still during that. Then, they give you narcotics, which slow down bowel motility, your bowels don't move as fast when you're on narcotics. And then, you get antibiotics that change the flora of your gut. And then you're asked to make this great recovery, but you're hurting because you have postoperative pain.
>
> So again, you're not moving much. You're static, and when you don't move, your bowels actually don't move. Going for a walk is the best thing you can do to help you go to the bathroom. So, these things all interrelate, and you're having multiple things affecting you. Having a good preoperative and postoperative diet can counteract a lot of these effects because you're getting your GI in a position where it's optimized, and you're going to be able to recover faster and more effectively from the insults that you're having as a result of surgery, which are opioids, stasis, meaning not moving around, and antibiotics."

Let's get back to that word, microbiome. Dr. Bruening helped to explain exactly what that means in nutritional terms. Dr. Bruening said:

I would definitely go for some foods that contain probiotics or are fermented because, if I'm going to have surgery, the doctors are going to give me antibiotics and that will damage my gut microbiome and I need it to grow back as fast as possible and I need it to grow back healthy. So, I would probably include . . . well, my personal favorites are yogurt. That's just a preference. But if I liked things like fermented vegetables and sauerkraut, I would be sure to eat those. At least a little bit every day or every other day, also.

Dr. Bruening continued:

I'm right now talking about the gut microbiome and some people call it the gut microbiota. But we have many, many, many millions of different kinds of bacteria that live in our intestinal tract, and what you eat can affect the composition of your gut microbiome in a very short time. There've been some very interesting studies that have shown that people with different types of diseases have very different gut microbiomes. For example, obese people have a very different composition in their gut microbiome than that of lean people.

You may have read some of the, I think shocking things about people with serious intestinal disease like Crohn's disease, getting a terrible intestinal infection called C DIFF, Clostridium difficile, which is miserable. It causes nonstop diarrhea, it's painful, and we don't have any good treatments for it. But one of the experimental treatments that's being done here and in other countries is fecal transplant. Basically, your feces are a good example of a gut microbiome. So, they take feces from a healthy person and transplant it into someone who has these terrible GI infections and, in some cases, they got some extremely miraculous and amazing recoveries.

Nutrition is a very new science. It's only been around for about 100 years. We've learned a lot. But there's still so much we don't know. So, we're just beginning to understand this. But what we do know, in adults, is that adults who eat probiotics, which are fermented foods, tend to have a healthier gut microbiome than people who do not eat those foods. Eating things like sugar and processed fats tends to favor the growth of the undesirable microbes in your gut, whereas eating the healthy foods that I've listed to you several times—the veggies, the fruits, the legumes, the nuts, the seeds, the whole grains—tends to favor the growth of the more healthy and favorable microbes in the microbiota. It's kind of like weeds in the garden. Do you want the good stuff to grow in your garden or do you want it to be overrun with weeds?

Bone broth has been shown to have some wonderful healing properties, and it tends to be rich in minerals in particular. Rebecca Katz, an integrative nutritionist and chef, has a recipe for what she calls Magic Mineral Broth[11], which is vegetarian-based mineral broth. I have

11. https://www.rebeccakatz.com/magic-mineral-broth/

> no idea how that would compare to an actual bone broth made from bones. We can assume that your gut microbiome would be damaged by the use of antibiotics. So, to regrow a healthy microbiome, what you would want to do is make sure that you're eating all those healthy plant-based foods I've listed—the veggies, the fruits, the legumes, the nuts, the whole grains, etc., etc., and you also want to include the fermented foods. They're almost, if I can make an analogy, almost like fertilizing the good bacteria in the gut that will give you a healthy microbiome, and staying away from the sugar, which will favor the growth of the less helpful microbes in the gut.

Robert G. added his point of view:

> And, I would say that I'm probably about the same weight, surprisingly, that I was prior to surgery now. And, it's taken me awhile to lose some, because I definitely gained some, I would say, in the first nine months. But, I think eating better the past eight months or so, is definitely helping me. And, once I get down to Mexico and eat that good food down there all the time it will be easier—everything's so much fresher. No more In-N-Out burgers down there.

It's a commitment to do the homework and the legwork to put this food strategy to work to give your body what it needs to give you the full recovery you are hoping for. That brings us to the final chapter of "Becoming You Again." Becoming an optimized patient is the key to the clinical success you want after enduring the rigor of a major and successful spine surgery. Does it work? Can you actually fire up your recovery engine? After years of struggle can you actually be you again? Everyone at the table thinks you can. Do you?

(Since the publication of this book I have created a nutrition-based meal plan featuring 60 original recipes focused on healing. Our methodology was to create a "field of nutrition with ingredients that aid healing" and then have a distinguished chef turn those ingredients into something wonderful to eat. If you have ever seen the show "Chopped" on the Food Network, you know that a gifted chef can make almost any combination of ingredients into something delicious to eat. Our theory was, if they can that for taste, we can do it for nutrition. The meal plan recipes are currently part of an interactive program created by Optimized Outcome Solutions, LLC[12]. We hope to release a cook book for general market consumption in 2022.)

12. www.OptimzedOutcome.com

12

BECOMING YOU AGAIN

If you are anything like all of the patients we have heard from, what you want from your surgery and recovery plan is to be you again—to be free of pain and to be able to do the things that you enjoy, that give your life meaning. I asked everyone what they most hoped for from their surgery. Among the half dozen of us quoted in this book, I want to start with Lucio D. He had a very simple and emotional concern. Lucio shared:

> The fact that I wasn't going to be able to look up in the sky and do it for a long time. The fact that now I'd have to be way leaned back in some sort of chair to look up at the night sky. And that was a huge fear. Of course, you can't do that after surgery, right? You can't do that for like a month after surgery. You just have to start practicing slowly and every day incrementally working yourself there.

Lucio brightened as he continued:

> So, now I can sit back, I can stand and look straight up and actually lean my head back. You know, not for

> a long, long time, but for a good half hour before I'm like, okay, this is getting uncomfortable. But I can still sit there and look up, and that was a huge fear of mine. I was like, oh no, I'm now limited in my movement, which is going to make me not be able to see those stars. It was just really dumb and it turned out to be nothing. Now I can look up, because I used it as a fear of "I don't want that to happen. What can I do?" And I even asked the doctor about "my rotation." He goes, "You can go as far as your body will let you. But just so you know, the more you stretch, the more you try incrementally without hurting yourself, you should be able to get a good angle on your neck." And I did, and it worked out fine. But, you know, there was a huge fear of that. I was sad over it for a while because I love looking up at the stars at night!

Each of us had a fear, a hope, and finally a goal. I start with Lucio because he didn't want to ski in the Olympics or return to cage fighting like Nathan Quarry, he just wanted to see the stars in the sky.

Having fully recovered from his fall off the mountain, Doug Amend had this observation:

> Again, the worst thing going into and coming out of the surgery was thinking that I wasn't gonna be able to do the things that I did before. That I was gonna have to resign myself to either no longer being able to play golf or no longer being able to play hockey or no longer being able to be physically able to do the things

> that I was doing. In my mind I was resigning myself to the fact that, well, I'm glad I enjoyed them while I did because I'm never going to be able to do them again, go snowboarding, for example, so just the recreational activities. I thought my recreational days were over. The conversation with Nathan (Quarry) is what turned that around. Even after surgery I was still resigning myself to the fact I wasn't gonna be able to do all this stuff. I might as well start selling my gear. And Nathan said, "Dude, it's just your back. It'll heal. You'll never think about it again." And I'm just like, "Even if you shut it down for six months?" Nathan said, "I can tell you it'll happen." Now after that time I can go, wow, he was 100% right!"

Doug, encouraged by Nathan Quarry, has fully recovered. He realized that by getting his mindset adjusted by Nate that he was able to become him again. Meaning, he was able to do all of the things that he feared would be part of his past not part of his future.

Joy H. offered a cautionary, but helpful, note about her road back to who she was. Joy said: "You manage your expectations, that's probably my biggest advice, post op." I then asked, "What's the one thing you would advise people?" She offered:

> Understanding the timeline we're operating on. It's not just, "We pulled a number out of a hat about how long it's going to take you to heal." Those are actually scientifically proven numbers. It takes between six months and two years for a bone to fuse, that kind of thing. My surgeon estimated it's probably going to be

> a year recovery for you, and I didn't take him at his word, and he was doing me a favor by saying that. I think we all think that the surgeon's going to exaggerate that number, or, "I'm young and I'm going to beat the odds." I get weird ideas about who I am and what I can achieve physically, and that wasn't realistic and it devastated me for a while there. Emotionally, it dragged me down, and that was not doing myself a favor, by being discouraged and depressed and things like that after surgery. That wasn't helping me physically, either, by battling depression.

Joy's recovery experience was so powerful for her that she now helps prospective spine patients find resources and patient ambassadors to help new patients have the best possible outcome. In fact, all of the patients who contributed their very personal medical experiences for this book are volunteers who regularly talk to people suffering with chronic back pain in an effort to help them understand the facts of what is entailed in spine surgery. Sadly, many patients fearing the "horror stories" of spine surgery are unwilling to make the commitment to recover and reclaim a pain-free life.

Robert G. struggled for years on the job in his automotive business before he committed to putting an end to his chronic pain. Hoping for a pain-free retirement in Mexico, he was willing to bet on himself and see the surgeon. His decision, like mine, like all of the decisions of all the patients in this book, was not without concern. Doug recalled, "That was my biggest fear: going through all of that and not having any kind of results at all." If I have learned anything from curating the interviews in this book it is that the horror stories of the past are exactly that, a thing of the past. I have also learned that so much of the outcome is in the patient's hands, and that if you have the right mindset and commitment, the chances are very good that you are going to have a good outcome.

Robert G. underlines this point of view:

> I felt it was such a success, of all the pain being gone right away, because he said it's very rare. It was, because I felt that the surgery was so successful, for me, of getting rid of the pain. And, the fear of going through that surgery, I think for me, not knowing for sure if the pain would go away, and that it did for me; I want to help other people understand that it can help. But, again, by the same token, everybody's different, and I don't want to get somebody's hopes up that it would work for everybody. But, just feeling how the surgery was so successful for me, to where I no longer have the pain—I was shocked at how well it did for me. I absolutely have not one bit of pain that I had before; I am able to do things that I was not able to do leading up to the surgery. My body wasn't able to function prior to that, that's correct, without having tears in my eyes. I just appreciate you giving me the opportunity to tell my story. Hopefully all the information helps and the key to it all is to help other people who have to go through it and to ease their mind and make the decision. And, just hope that other people have as much success as I had.

I asked Dr. Sanjay Khurana to summarize how he saw the role of surgery in helping patients to "become you again." We spoke directly about the patient's role in that goal. Dr. Khurana said:

> Surgery is a clinical tool to address certain structural deficiencies in the body so the rest of the body can carry on. We're really just helping the body heal. In some instances, major trauma, and so forth, it's not generally elective surgery, it's really just corrective surgery. But, in a lot of what we do we're trying to do exactly what you said, shepherd a way for the body to function the way it was designed to function. The one thing that's pretty progressive, I think, in society now, is that longevity is becoming a more common phenomenon. We're living much longer and longer and that's a testament to public health, to intervention, to our heart doctors, to immunizations, and so forth. But, by the same token, I think that our ability to correct the mechanical parts that continue to age has not caught up to the same extent that our longevity has. So over time, especially in an aging population, we're going to see much more opportunity for limited surgical intervention to play a role in optimizing patients.

It is important to hear Dr. Khurana's point that over time, wear and tear is going to occur especially as we live longer and longer. It is interesting to note his reference to "optimizing patients." Along the way of formulating this book, the doctors immediately connected with this concept. Becoming you again is just the last phase of the optimized patient process. For those of you who are still on the fence, consider the scope and confidence of Dr. Khurana's statement. He is seeing hundreds of patients who have freed themselves from chronic pain and have been restored to normal function. Dr. Khurana humorously circled back to the challenge found in mindset and patient expectations. He said:

> In terms of outcome, I think it's very important to correlate an outcome with a patient expectation. So, if someone is extraordinarily debilitated and in a wheelchair, I think sometimes, the joke is, the patient will say, "Well, can I golf after surgery?" Then the trick question is, "Well, do you golf now?" And the patient says, "No. I've never golfed in my life."

It's a joke, but there is a very serious truth within it. I am not exactly the way I was before my car accident. However, I no longer need to use catheters six times a day, I no longer need to take three different medications, I no longer have lower back and leg pain, I no longer need to take an over-the-counter pain pill every few hours. Am I me again? Not exactly, but I am getting closer to the best possible outcome by daily and consciously trying to improve my gait. I still have reduced function in my calves and it interferes with my gait. And by the way, on a scale of 1 to 10, 1 being limping and 10 being a perfect gait, I have improved from a 1 before surgery to a 9. Skycaps at airports no longer race to aid me with a wheelchair. And by the way, I never allowed them to put me in a wheelchair, no matter how much it hurt. I preferred to walk on my way to getting better.

Dr. Khurana expanded on my thought:

> You've really got to find a realistic goal based on the age, the morbidity, the intrinsic mobility, as well as other issues. So, for example, if we fix someone's back from a claudication and nerve standpoint, they may still have bone on bone on their hips, they may still have bone on bone in their knee, they may still have other issues, so you can't necessarily optimize a patient looking at the patient as one organ. I think the benefit of being a spine surgeon is that, oftentimes, we have to by design look at other segments in the body, whether its joints, any inflammatory conditions, we have to take that into the overall outcome. The unfortunate reality is a lot of patients with spine pathology tend to have other musculoskeletal issues such as degenerative knees and degenerative, arthritic hips and ankles, and so forth.

Dr. Khurana's reference to bone on bone knee issues is not random. He sent me to see the knee specialist as the physical therapists were working on my gait. It turned out that his review of my films showed bone on bone osteoarthritis in my right knee. Dr. Khurana referred me to a knee specialist. And, yes, I optimized for that surgery. Without any hype it was astonishing to the knee surgeon and my physical therapist how quickly and fully I healed. I know it may sound like I am a train wreck, but truly, I am doing just fine.

Dr. Khurana continues:

> So, given this day and age of specialty care where you have a knee replacement expert, and a hip replacement expert, and foot and ankle, a spine, a sports, everything

is so super fragmented, I do feel that it is one of my obligations to kind of be the cruise director and tell people, listen, we're going to fix this, but then you gotta see a hip person, you gotta see a urologist or whatever. Try to get everything in order, because I feel like from the spine down we kind of control all these segments from mobility and although I'm not the guy who will replace the joints or do the sports medicine, I do feel I have the ability to at least orchestrate where those pieces will fit into the long-term picture. In terms of expectations, I think one thing is really just to get a sense of their functional station and get a sense of where they expect themselves to be. If the expectation is a fairly simple one, which is like, 'I have this nerve pain in my leg and I really want it to go away,' that's a relatively simple expectation. That's a fairly simple thing that we can fix by taking the pressure off the nerve. If the expectation is that, 'I don't want any back pain whatsoever,' then it's my job to temper those expectations down and say, 'Listen, we can treat the most significant nerve compression, but the ability for a simple surgery to take all the back pain that you've had for the past ten years away, may not be realistic."

What is realistic for you is something that you must ask your surgeon before you sign the pre-op order.

Dr. Branko agreed with Dr. Khurana but cautioned about my high hopes for this book. Dr. Branko said, "You're not gonna reach everybody, but every patient that you can reach and every patient that you can help, that otherwise wouldn't have been helped, is a massive accomplishment. What you're doing is great. I like it." It is ironic that one of the first people I reached with the *The Optimized Patient* approach wasn't even a spine patient. I have talked a lot about my dumb luck of bumping into the right people just when I needed them. A screenwriting buddy of mine here in Hollywood has the same dumb luck I have because he knows me! Adam, who I have mentioned several times in earlier chapters, was considering having a deviated septum fixed which was causing him breathing problems. Over the past couple of years, he has observed me getting injured, going through several surgeries, and then recovering. He also noted that along the way of fixing my back problems, that I had also become a lot leaner. Adam is, in truth, one of the smartest people I know. There are few subjects that Adam does not have some in-depth knowledge about or some arcane fact associated with it. So, he was very interested in hearing what I was learning about surgery and the role of mindset, rest, and nutrition in my recovery. I asked Adam if he would like to share his experience in a book about the process we both benefitted from and he enthusiastically said yes. Adam recalls,

> You and I have been friends for a long time, and I'd noticed that you had, you know, both lost weight and were looking really good and you had talked about the underlying philosophy which was that you could prepare your body for surgery so that it would respond in the best possible manner. And I'd already made a determination that I wanted to take care of a couple of small

> surgeries, at this point in my life, rather than a decade or two decades from now. And I thought anything I can do to help make that process more successful, I wanted to try if it made sense. It made sense to me on a couple of levels. If you can take the stress off your system, and I'm sure I could eat steak and hamburgers and go to McDonalds and not die, at least immediately, it occurred to me that all those things put stress on your system, and that any energy your system was expending on that stress was energy it wasn't expending on helping you heal the most efficaciously. I also happen to like vegetables, so for me the hardest part was giving up sugar—and I've been known to eat a barbecue or two—and enjoy it. But I thought, I'll make a commitment to this.

I would like to share with you that this conversation took place long before Dr. Bruening had directed me to the Harvard MyPlate. Adam articulates well both the commitment and the common-sense necessity of eating things that help rather than hinder recovery. After his doctor told Adam that his rate and quality of healing was certainly in the top 1% of patients, Adam was already well on his way to being the best Adam he could be. Common sense dictated, in the larger scheme of things, that as long as the optimized plan worked for his surgery, why not for the rest of his life? Adam concluded:

> Surgery by definition is traumatic; somebody's opening up your body which is normally a closed system. It is a trauma, I think surgeons call it an insult, and your body must recover from that insult and that trauma,

> and anything you can do to help your body accomplish that is a good thing. I think it's effective not just for that but as an overall, you know, way of life. I would recommend anybody who tries this that you'll find that you will be doing it long after the surgery's done because it just works really well, makes you feel good, your energy's good, you know, you find yourself losing weight and your friends are, "Oh, Adam you look good!"

The comedian in Adam couldn't resist quipping, "I don't know, you may wanna clean your glasses." Several months after I formally interviewed Adam, he reported to me that he is continuing to eat a mostly vegetarian diet that is consistent with the Harvard MyPlate. He was delighted to note that he is continuing to lose weight while increasing his energy.

I end with Adam to make clear that it would appear that an effort to optimize works for any kind of surgery patient. My experience in the widest possible context of recovering from trauma is applicable to anybody who needs the help of a surgeon to heal their body. As I developed the outline and approach for this book, I believed I knew what I wanted to say about helping people to be optimized patients. After my imaginary dinner party, my understanding of *The Optimized Patient* idea was somewhat different than my original thoughts. Here, in summary, is what I learned, with you, from the good people who shared their fears, their hopes, and their triumphs for this book.

The doctors, who I presumed would be focused on the physical condition of the patients, were equally concerned about the patients' mindset. The "will to get well" really is the essential first step to optimizing for the surgery. If you don't believe you can get well, it is unlikely that you will take the actions necessary to accomplish getting well. This realization brings me back, again, to the first words of this book "it's a commitment." Your commitment to get well is an expression of your will to get well and stay well.

It was also unexpected to learn how influential patient expectations are in the optimized patient preparation scenario. Interestingly, your expectations are constantly in play with your will to get well. If your expectations are that you expect to be immediately pain free, your dream may come true as it did with Robert G. But, if you are not 100% yourself again in the time frame the doctor has anticipated, the process of recovery can begin to feel like a defeat rather than a victory. One of the ways to regain and sustain a positive mindset is to make sure that you celebrate all wins—no matter how small. Each of the patients who contributed their story to this book recovered over a long period of time. Several of them, including me, are still in an ongoing effort to regain function, restore gait, or just look up at the stars. As we learned from each of the surgeons, a clinical failure can follow a perfect surgery if the patient isn't compliant and active in their own recovery. This view was confirmed by our two physical therapists who stressed that proper guidance in your recovery is essential to an optimized outcome. For those of you who are skeptical and may think the physical therapists are feathering their own nest, believe me they are not. Nothing will ruin a perfect recovery faster than pushing yourself beyond what is appropriate, manageable pain into the arena of damaging pain.

Despite all of the negative press about the use and overuse of opioids, the doctors and physical therapists were definite that pain relievers play a critical role in successful recovery. As we discussed, the key is to be willing to use less and less painkiller as your healing progresses. Rest is a fundamental part of any healing process no matter if it's healing from surgery or getting over the flu. Bed rest is a time-honored aspect of getting well. The key role that opioids play in rehab, we learned, was to ensure that you can get comfortable enough to get quality rest. But, the press reports are right; the opioids pose an addiction risk. You will be happy to know that opioids only pose an addiction risk when the patient continues to take them after the pain could be well managed with over-the-counter products. Said simply, if Aleve or Advil will do the job, put the prescriptions away!

The combination of anesthesia to put you to sleep, antibiotics to protect against infection, and opioids to manage pain has massive and unintentional consequences on your gut health. The importance of your microbiome (a word I learned long after my first surgery) cannot be overstated. I believe everyone understands that our bodies need to be nourished to heal. What most of us likely do not know is that after surgery the anesthesia, antibiotics and opioids have shut down your gut, which is the gateway to nourishing your body for healing. Increasingly, the medical community is embracing the idea that if your gut it not optimized, your ability to absorb the nourishment you need to heal is diminished. I wish I could expand Chapter 11 further with respect to proper nutrition before and after surgery. Truly, that would be—should be—a book in itself. Special thanks to Dr. Kay Bruening at Syracuse University for sharing resources that provide both insight and recipes to help your gut health recover as quickly as possible. Beyond becoming you again, good nutrition is a part of the optimized strategy that may actually serve you for the rest of your life.

If you have read Chapter 11 closely and taken the time to look at the current understanding on MyPlate from Harvard University, you will have noticed activity plays a significant role in healthy living. In the lower left hand corner, you will see a graphic representation of a person running, with the exclamatory call to action "Stay Active!" The information contained in this image holds the keys to giving your body the nourishment it needs to heal. As we learned from the surgeons, the sooner you are up on your feet and moving, the better. Working with a physical therapist to safely ratchet up your activity without injury is another key ingredient to being an optimized patient. And, don't forget to ask your physical therapist about how you can use a swimming pool to optimize your prehab and your rehab.

Dr. Vermon Esplin provide a final insight from his 30-years of helping patients to recover function and relieve pain,

> I'm good friends with a number of orthopedists, and there's a total joint surgeon who's very active and very busy. Right now, the trend is going to outpatient total joint surgery and total knees and total hips. An important part of the person being able to go home the same day as they have their total knee and total hip is the preoperative counseling and level of expectations. You obviously, have to choose the right patients that don't have a lot of health problems and are going to be on

> that far end of the Bell curve that we talked about who are motivated and want to recover quickly. But a lot of that is helping them to understand what's expected, what process to go through, and what to do, and when to do it.

I am going to give our mountaineer, Doug Amend, the final quote about why he feels so moved to contribute to this book. Doug's response was immediate and heartfelt:

> I want to help. I can give them what Nathan gave me, 100% confident information. I've been there. I've done this. You can do it. Here's how it works. No surprises. I don't think the future looks any different than had I not fallen off the mountain. I mean, my perspective today is that the mountain was an adventure that I had. I've had other adventures in my life, but I'm back to being Dougie. I just do what I do, behave like I behave, and the injury, the surgery, doesn't define me. People who meet me who know it happened, they just shake their head. They say I would have never expected you to be out on the ice, up on the mountain, stuff like that. That's amazing. And the people I meet for the first time, they have no clue what I went through.

Your health truly is your wealth. If I learned anything on this journey from talking to the patients, doctors, physical therapists, chiropractors, and nutritionists it is this: successfully preparing for, surviving, and recovering from spine surgery is really in your control. The key ingredient is your will to get well and your willingness to do the hard work of healing. Like I said in the first line of this book, if you want to get well, it's a commitment.

If you've made the commitment to read this book, you definitely have what it takes to be you again. The only thing that separates you from the life you are dreaming about and praying for is your willingness to finish the job that the surgeons have started for you as an optimized patient.

ADDENDUM FOR CAREGIVERS

This addendum was initiated by patient Doug Amend after he read the first draft of this book. He was of the opinion that The Optimized Patient *wasn't complete without giving some guidance to caregivers. He was right on target. To the caregivers who are reading this special section, please forgive your patient, for they know not what they are doing. As you will learn in this brief addition, the only thing that is as hard as being a spine patient is being the poor soul who is taking care of them. My thanks to Doug Amend for his contribution.*

As we have learned, spine surgery is a scary option to consider. There are so many questions, so much information, so many discussions, and so many possible outcomes. For the patient, the pain you are dealing with is amplified by the unknown of "Will I be better or worse?" We've looked at the doctor's role in answering those questions and optimizing the patient to get through it. Just as important as your surgeon, your caregiver(s) has a critical role to play in your best recovery. Your caregiver is another angle (and angel) that should not be overlooked. Your spouse, kids, brother, sister, or friends probably have as many questions and concerns as you do. I'd like to offer some insight into the caregiver side of the equation because **after surgery you are going to be a whole different person when you get wheeled out of the operating room.**

The big note the patients and caregivers get from the surgeon is no BLT for months. No, that's not a sandwich. It's no Bending, Lifting or Twisting. If you are a caregiver, and if this is the only part of this book that you are reading, think about life without BLT. Prepare yourself to deal with a loved-one in pain who is challenged with every aspect of the activities of daily living: walking to the bathroom, being able to hold it until they get there, using the bathroom unassisted, showering, dressing themselves, cooking, and feeding themselves. Assuming you are a caregiver living with or assisting someone close to you who is now considering spine surgery to relieve pain and/or increase mobility, I would like to share my experience in the hopes of helping you achieve a successful outcome too. I am 100% convinced my wife, as caregiver, was both completely unprepared for, yet totally instrumental in my successful recovery.

This is the part that I feel requires illumination as part of the successful clinical outcome. The team you have in place would benefit from understanding the combined effects from spine surgery. It starts with the appointments. As the caregiver you are along for the ride making sure all of the questions are asked and answered. As the caregiver you help with the medications and exercises before choosing surgery. Once surgery becomes the chosen option, you again attend the appointments to keep track of the questions. You do your best to understand and support. You make preparations at home for recovery. You plan to prepare the meals for recovery. You do your best to understand the overall time frame for being in the hospital, being off work, going to physical therapy, and estimating the time needed for getting back to 100%.

Nurses and occupational therapists at the hospital outlined, before discharge, things like how to set up the home, what items are useful to have, and recommended taking a walker home a day early to test moving it through the hallways and doorways. My wife, Michelle, offered her number one recommendation to any spine patient, "Ask for help, and graciously accept the help that is offered." The key problem here is that those who offer help really do not know what to do or what help you need. Michelle added, "I finally figured out that by giving a small task to each person who asked to help, something to do—my day was much better." A couple examples she shared was inviting one of my buddies over for lunch. After preparing a couple of sandwiches she now had a couple of hours for herself while we played poker. I was entertained. She had a neighbor do a weekly grocery run for staples. She had my dad call each day and talk for 30 minutes or so at the same time. This allowed her to take a shower, knowing I would not try to get up and take care of myself.

To help me get in and out of bed, she successfully identified the "log roll" method a couple of days after straining her back. Since I slept on my back I was instructed by her to raise my knees and pull my feet up to my bottom. I was then to rotate my whole body (not twisting) with my knees hanging over the edge of the bed. Finally, I would extend my feet off the bed and in one motion roll up to the sitting position. This required her to help with my head and shoulders, letting my feet hit the floor. Unfortunately, she did not find this preferred method until the second or third day. For the first couple of days she was doing her absolute best to "lift" me up to the sitting position. I outweigh her by a good 50 pounds and this strained her back. Good information, but a little late.

The challenge of taking a shower is both mechanical and emotional. Not being able to wash my lower body, again no Bend, Lift or Twist, seems mechanical. In my reality it was emotional too. "Seriously? I cannot even wash myself?" This began to impact my mental state. A long handle sponge purchased at the hospital gift shop was hugely beneficial once I was able to shower by myself. Standing outside of the shower afterwards and not knowing how hard to pat someone dry led to the discovery of a large beach towel. All that was needed was to drape the towel over my head and shoulders. Just wrapping my arms allowed for most of the water to quickly be soaked up.

Driving, or better yet, not driving, also was more mental for me. It irritated me not to drive. I usually drove everywhere. I drove her everywhere I could. I helped drive others, and now I was relegated to being chauffeured. While this in itself does lend to being a "First World" problem, it is the stacking or layering effect that will ultimately cause poor behavior later. My daughter, bless her heart, researched and demanded I apply for a Temporary Handicap Parking Placard. I was not a fan. I yielded, because it was winter, because it was icy, and because she wanted to protect me from having to walk any distance in a back brace in bad weather. Beautiful girl. Mentally, though, it just piled another layer on me.

Harvey asked my surgeon, Dr. Anthony Hadden, to comment on what caregivers need to know, from the surgeon's perspective, about the patient's condition after exiting the operating room. Dr. Hadden shared, "You also have to understand how pain affects the mind. Doug is a stoic guy. He fell off a mountain, broke his back, hiked out of the mountain for 9 hours, or whatever the heck it was, and then shows up at the emergency room because he looked like crap and his wife made him go—and then talks his way out of even staying at the hospital. Pain is still going to rear its head and show up in different ways. **In some people, it's their nice-ability factor—they become irritable, cantankerous."**

The medicine started with the opioid painkiller. Needed, definitely needed. Rest is critical and hard to come by when in pain. My wife started a notebook and tracked every dose she administered. She followed the surgeon's orders to the letter. Unfortunately, there were no muscle relaxers prescribed at discharge from the emergency room. The surgeon thought they had been prescribed and was surprised when we reached out four days later before our appointment for more painkillers. Dr. Hadden said, "You shouldn't need any more. Are you taking the muscle relaxers?" We did not have any. Dr. Hadden responded immediately, "OMG, I will call them in. Can you head over now?" Double check the meds with the doctor if you are not seeing the pain relief as promised.

My mood change was definitely a marriage tester. Michelle shared, "I now know it was temporary. However, at the time, the severity of the mood change was noticeable. I wasn't sure if it was from the painkillers, the anesthesia, the actual incident, or what? Doug was different. He was abrupt and kind of unpleasant. His diet was smaller, only wanted bland foods. I felt the painkillers altered his behavior, but I did not know for sure. It did not matter to me. Even though I felt really underappreciated I was grateful I had him."

Dr. Hadden had something to add here, "I tell that to patients all the time and their families, especially when they are in the room, I say, 'Look, you're going to have pain. You are not going to be a nice person to be around. And the family member usually pipes up and says, 'Yeah, they are really not nice to be around.' Dealing with this pain chronically definitely affects you psychologically."

Not being able to do anything, literally, was difficult. I was either in bed, in a chair, or in the way. Getting in and out of a chair was no cakewalk. Again, Michelle speed-researched and found we could rent a stand-up chair. The one for old folks. Here we go again with the mental state. We had it delivered and it was fantastic. Made a huge difference being able to launch right into my walker after surgery. The mental dismantling of masculinity continued. I was quarantined to the first floor of our home for 30 days with instructions not to leave the house. And, I was bored.

Dr. Hadden gave us some insight into the role pain plays in the post-operative experience. Dr. Hadden said, "Pain is a significant problem, and we try to deal with that as best as we can, but, all we conceptually think of is the physical action of the pain, but we are not thinking of the psychological aspect of the pain. There are two separate pathways for pain, what is called the lateral pathway and the medial pathway. The lateral pathway is, I hit my finger with a hammer and it hurts like hell. The medial pathway is, I hit my finger with hammer and, man, now I am depressed about it and really mad at myself because I hit my finger with the hammer.

That's the emotional aspect. Most people, and physicians in particular, treat the lateral pathway, the actual pain, rather than the psychological portion."

As a caregiver, you are busting your backside to provide support. You also have your life to maintain. Worse, you are preparing meals, fluffing pillows, administering medication, helping your loved ones in and out of chairs, beds, cars, and the like, only to be dismissed or yelled at. Who would do that? Sadly, the hurting bird you are taking care of will. Not intentionally. Not even consciously. The combination of the injury, the surgery, the recovery, the pain medication, and lack of activity combine to temporarily alter the personality. Personally, I was not that pleasant to be around. After the surgery I was sore and uncomfortable. Despite her over-the-top efforts I struggled to be appreciative. At first she was sympathetic. As time wore on, I wore on her. About three weeks after surgery I got up from my chair and worked my walker to the front door. It had snowed the night before and was still snowing that morning. As the snow piled up on our driveway my wife bundled up and pulled our snow-blower out of the garage. She wanted the driveway clear for our other daughter to be able to come over. I watched as she struggled to blow the snow off the driveway. Instead of being appreciative, I opened the door and barked at her that she was doing it wrong. Right? What the hell was wrong with me? She continued on and eventually my neighbor, who had been religiously shoveling our driveway for three weeks, came over and finished. He then let me know not to worry about the driveway. It was his way of politely telling me not to talk to her that way. He was no better prepared to deal with me. He wanted to be sympathetic, yet knew that I was a burden to her.

One of the areas I experienced where information is lacking is understanding the behavior of a spine patient on opioids. No one prepared my wife for my behavior. Being sent home in a back brace with a prescription for opioid painkillers and instructions to not bend, lift or twist until an appointment the following week forced her to do speed research on "How to care for someone with a broken back?" There were many challenges: I needed help getting in and out of bed, I needed help taking a shower, I could no longer drive because I was on painkillers and not able to twist, I was on a pain management regimen of opioids that required scheduled intake, I needed help getting in and out chairs. I was bored out of my mind and in the way of daily household life. Harvey shared with me that his wife, Wileen, was present with him at his discharge. He was so looped on the anesthesia and painkillers that he completely mis-remembered the discharge instructions. Had Wileen not been present to hear the instructions and guide Harvey in the process, he might have made a serious mistake with his pain meds.

At the beginning, and certainly during, caregiving is a thankless job. You gladly commit the time and energy to see your spouse, family member, or friend recover.

What was never shared with us was just what a challenging journey this would be.

Once you are in, there is really no option to stop. And when the opioid medication, boredom, soreness combine to ruin your patient's day—you are the nearest target. I have apologized, several times, for the incidents I remember. I do my best to apologize for the ones I don't remember too.

Meeting with a surgeon is a stressful experience. This list will help make sure you cover all the bases:

1. What are the risks and complications associated with the procedure?
2. How long will the patient be in the hospital post-operation?
3. What level of pain can the patient expect following the operation and how will it be managed?
4. Will the patient need any durable medical equipment following surgery for the home (i.e., walker, cane, crutches, toilet riser, shower chair, or lift chair)?
5. Should the patient follow a specific diet before or after surgery?
6. What should be my role in helping the patient shower after surgery?
7. What is the proper way to care for the incision(s)?
8. If a back brace is to be worn, at what times and for how long?
9. What should I be prepared to do with regard to getting the patient in and out of bed and making him or her comfortable?
10. What should be my time commitment during the recovery process?

One last list of ideas that I hope will be helpful. Your doctor may give you this kind of information, but not all do. For the sake of your patient, prepare your home prior to surgery.

11. Clear walkways by removing rugs and cords, and rearranging furniture if necessary
12. Move commonly used items to easy-to-reach places (waist level and above)
13. Prepare and freeze meals for at least the first week post-operation
14. Consider preparing a room or location on the first floor for the patient to sleep
15. Secure stair railings
16. Have slip-on shoes with non-skid soles readily available
17. Place skid-resistant strips in the bathtub
18. Have loose and comfortable clothing easily accessible
19. Prepare any medical equipment recommended by the surgeon so that it is ready-to-use, typically a walker
20. Large beach towels work best for drying after showers
21. Having a long shoe horn and a mechanical grabber will help the patient feel empowered
22. Request a surgeon's note to obtain a Temporary Handicap Parking Permit

You will receive specific discharge information that includes what to be aware of if something is going wrong. Read all instructions and be vigilant in watching for trouble signs. The life of the person in your charge may depend on it.

I gladly take care of my wife with no expectations. It is what I signed up for over 37 years ago. But to me, the surgical experience seemed different–above and beyond. Not everyone's experiences will be the same. I may have been at the low end of the spectrum with my behavior, but I have seen no benchmarks to gauge against. Even so, I believe that recognizing and preparing the caregiver will pay dividends for all who read this book. My contribution to *The Optimized Patient* is helping you to optimize your recovery team. If we have learned anything from creating this book it is that healing from spine surgery is a team sport and everyone's role is critically important if you want the outcome to be optimized.

AFTERWORD

by Nathan "Rock" Quarry

Nathan "Rock" Quarry is a retired American mixed martial arts fighter who is most notable for his appearance in The Ultimate Fighter, *a reality show from the Ultimate Fighting Championship, and for co-hosting the show* MMA Uncensored Live.

"I'm not getting surgery. I don't need surgery. I'm NOT getting surgery. The Doc is going to give me some oral medications to take. Or I'll get some physical therapy. At worst I'll need an injection of some magical elixir. But I'm NOT getting surgery."

That's what I was thinking mere moments before my doctor told me I needed surgery. And even worse, a spinal fusion.

"Do you have any questions?" is inevitably the next sentence spoken by the Doctor who seems a little rushed and is behind by a half an hour already.

"Um... no," is the response. And of course it is. Because the Patient is in shock. After looking at the potential surgical schedule there's the wander back through the parking lot, the drive home, the tasteless meal, the TV being blankly stared at and at 2:00 AM, questions. Never-ending questions. Will it hurt? Will it work? Do I really need it? What are the odds of success? If I ask my doctor for other patients to talk to with that upset him/her? What's my recovery time? What are the side effects? What's the worst case/best case scenario?

And there are a couple more questions I didn't think to ask myself in the wee hours of the night, like how do I prepare for surgery and how do I best recover from surgery?

And when I would call the doctor's office with these questions the response I would receive was always proceeded with the phrase, "What we've seen in our office..." or "Most patients experience..."

It was never, "MY experience."

If you want to know what surgery is like, ask me. I've had eight. Through my own trial and error I've discovered what works, what doesn't and how best to prepare for surgery.

Oh how wonderful it would be if a visit to the Doctor involved waving a magic wand around and curing all that ails us. But that's not real life. The doctor sets us up to heal, puts our bodies in alignment and removes things that shouldn't be there. After that, it's up to us. Individually and with the help of those around us.

Once my Surgeon did his part, I did mine. And my journey to recovery culminated fifteen months later with my comeback fight shown live on Spike TV in the UFC. Just know that journey started just like every journey does, with a single step. Stepping away from my hospital bed. Taking steps down the hospital hallway. Taking steps when I got back home.

Taking ownership of my recovery. Doing my part.

You're now on your way to becoming an Optimized Patient. Listen to your doctor. Listen to your Therapist. Listen to those that have come before you. And oh so importantly, listen to your own body.

While on that road to recovery, don't be afraid to dream big, to set some lofty goals. You want to work in the garden again? You want to fix your car? You want to pick up your grandkids? You want to return to work? Even if that work is as a professional MMA fighter?

Go ahead and set goals. I did and I was able to achieve every last one of them.

–Nathan "Rock" Quarry

Index

A

Accepting the surgical fix 30, 61, 66–68, 72, 80

Accountability 18, 162, 172

Acupuncturist 60

Addiction (opioid) 164–167, 208

Aerobic conditioning 60, 102, 110, 210

Alignment (spinal) 53, 63, 65, 89, 100, 162, 224

Alternative (treatments) 49, 51, 67, 71, 100

Amend, Doug (patient) 8, 19, 20, 26, 34, 37-41, 45, 46, 53-55, 64, 115, 130, 143–145, 158–159, 165, 188, 197–199, 210, 213, 217

Amend, Michelle (caregiver) 215, 217, 218

American Institute for Cancer Research 184, 185

Anesthesia 8, 9, 136, 137, 140, 143, 179, 209, 217, 220

Antibiotics 8, 9, 136, 143, 179, 190, 192, 209

Aqua (therapy) 31, 32, 49, 51, 55, 67, 103, 104, 135, 152

Atrophy 27, 88, 91, 135

B

Bacteria (good) 191, 193

Bathroom 25, 46, 143, 166, 214

Bethanacol 10

Bicycle 16, 45, 163

Biome (micro) 188

Biomechanical 62, 63

Bluezones (Healthy diet) 185

Bowel (movements) 136, 143, 179

Broth (bone) 192

Bruening, Kay 179–181, 183–185, 190, 191, 206, 209

Buettner, Daniel 185

C

Cage fighting 144, 146, 223

Candidate (for surgery) 83, 85, 86, 88, 92, 96, 101, 117, 127

Cardio conditioning 107, 116, 188

Caregiver (caregiving) 130, 144, 213, 214, 216, 219, 220, 222

Carragee, Eugene (psychological profiles) 74

Catabolic 137, 138

Celebrate all wins 147, 148, 166, 208

Cervical disk 25, 100

Chiropractic, chiropractor 13, 17, 21, 47, 49, 51-53, 57, 61-65, 111, 211

Chronic pain 1, 12, 23, 33, 41, 47, 58, 68, 76, 82, 85, 199, 201, 218

Claudication (trouble walking) 26, 202

Clinical outcome (success, failure) 79, 85, 86, 103, 134, 140, 173, 180, 193, 208, 214

Clostridium 191

Coach, coaching 11, 18, 32, 115, 146, 147, 164, 176, 188

Collapsed disk 27, 88

Commitment, committed 1–4, 12, 16, 18, 32, 47, 72, 78, 81, 86, 95, 97, 106, 108, 111, 112, 117, 127, 133, 140, 142, 147, 156, 157, 160, 162, 164–166, 169, 172–174, 180, 193, 199, 206, 207, 211, 220, 221

Complication 93

Compressed, compression (nerves) 13, 27, 40, 88-92, 100, 204

Condition 16, 27, 30, 45, 46, 56, 68, 77, 88, 89, 92, 106, 108, 124, 126, 170, 171, 196, 207, 217

Conditioning 6, 13, 15, 16, 34, 56, 60, 102, 107, 110, 128, 210

Conditions 60, 102, 103, 110, 190, 202, 210

Considering (surgery) 1, 12, 13, 15, 56, 66, 72, 73, 78, 80, 96, 122, 168, 204, 214

Constipation 9, 137, 142, 143, 164, 179

Constriction (nerve) 27, 88, 90

Cortisone (shots) 22, 57

D

Decisions (important re: surgery) 13, 14, 17, 32, 63, 66, 75, 78, 80, 95, 98, 124, 126, 127, 171, 172, 199, 200

Decompression (nerve) 89, 90, 97, 98, 124, 125

Deficiencies 110, 137, 177, 200

Degenerative (disk disease) 20–22, 24, 27, 45, 67, 83, 88, 89, 98, 190, 203

Depression 74, 77, 144, 158, 161, 170, 198, 218

Device (medical) 1, 14, 31, 74, 106, 113

Diabetes 7, 178, 189

Diet, nutrition 17, 46, 117, 119, 176, 177, 180, 183–185, 187, 188, 207, 217, 221

Digestion related 9, 118, 178

Disc disease 20–22, 45, 57, 67, 83

Discectomy 27, 63, 134

Doctor-speak 124

Drinking alcohol 116, 118, 177, 184, 186

Drive (vehicle) 23, 24, 41, 42, 216, 220, 223

Drugs (good) 7, 9, 10

Drugs (side effects) 10, 58, 69, 72, 81, 165, 189

Duke University Sports Medicine 20

Dysfunction 27, 76, 88, 91

E

Eastern medicine 62

Educate the patient 32, 113, 114, 128, 167

Emergency (room, procedures) 8, 19, 37, 39, 70, 101, 210, 217

Energy 46, 176, 205, 207, 220

Epidural 13, 51, 53, 57, 61, 65, 123

ERAS (Enhanced Recovery After Surgery) 136, 142

Exercise (importance of) 12, 21, 22, 44, 52, 55, 56, 60, 78, 104, 105, 109, 110, 114, 115, 119, 134, 135, 141, 152, 153, 155, 158, 161, 163, 164, 187, 188, 214

Experimental treatments 191

F

Failure (clinical) 79, 80, 86, 107, 140, 173, 208

Family support 130, 131, 162, 170, 218, 220
Fatty fish 182
Fear (fear related) 1, 14, 18, 67, 69, 78, 82, 121, 150, 195, 196, 198, 199
Fecal transplant 191
Fermented (foods) 190–193
Food (for healing) 3, 9–11, 13, 17, 24, 48, 159, 174–176, 178–182, 184, 186, 187, 189, 190, 192, 193, 217
Foramen (nerves) 98, 125
Four-part understanding 11
Fruit 175, 177, 178, 180, 182, 184, 185, 192, 193
Fuse 9, 14, 15, 20, 27, 40, 43, 45, 74, 76, 89, 90, 97–100, 124–126, 134, 145, 149, 198, 223

G

Gait dysfunction 88, 133, 135, 166, 172, 202, 203, 208
Galloway, Noah 161
Gastrointestinal 142, 179
Goals (goal setting) 18, 95, 157, 162, 225
Grain, grains 184, 185, 192, 193
Greens 116, 186
Grocery (for healing) 11–13, 176, 182, 215
Guidance to caregivers 213
Guidebook 1, 133, 168

H

Hadden, Anthony 39, 40, 54, 216–218
Hardware (surgical) 9, 14, 74
Harvard Healthy Eating Plate 181, 182, 187, 206, 207, 209
High-fructose corn syrup 190
High-quality protein 185
Hills, Christopher 30, 60, 78, 86, 87, 95–97, 101, 102, 109, 111, 116, 124, 125, 137, 138, 140, 142, 147, 173, 186, 196, 210
Hippocrates 10, 178
Honey, Manuka 136, 151, 183
Horror stories (Surgical) 13, 15, 29, 67, 68, 72, 73, 75–78, 80, 81, 83, 85, 92, 125, 132, 199
Hoyer Lifts 155
Hydrated, hydration 185
Hydrocodone 70
Hyperextension 106
Hypertension 7

I

Ibuprofen 19, 21, 38, 52
Incision 2, 3, 9, 106, 109, 146, 151, 221
Infection 53, 191, 209
Inflammation 31, 59, 113, 146
Inflammatory 108, 190, 202
Ingredients (needed for optimal outcome) 12, 140, 146
Injection 58, 82, 223
Injury 3, 10, 13, 19, 24–26, 31, 32, 38–40, 46, 48, 54, 72, 87, 91, 104, 112–114, 128, 133, 135, 151, 153, 154, 157, 158, 168, 178, 204, 210, 211, 219
Instability 27, 88–90, 98, 125
Instrumentation 89, 125, 126, 134
Insurance 1, 61, 62, 107, 112

Internet 29, 40, 49, 51, 63–66, 68, 80, 122
Intervention (surgical, pharmaceutical, etc) 7, 39, 63, 66, 73, 75, 78, 127, 146, 158, 201
Intestines 9, 191
Invasive, invasiveness (degrees of) 73–75, 83, 93, 126, 142

J

Joint (trauma, health) 31, 62, 63, 104, 105, 112, 113, 154, 167, 190, 202, 203
Joseph, Solomon (PT) 31, 32, 55, 56, 61, 65, 103, 104, 105, 134, 135, 152, 153, 154, 155, 172
Joy H. (patient, violinist) 23, 24, 41, 42, 44, 45, 59, 60, 65, 80, 97, 115, 118, 119, 120, 131, 148, 149, 150, 160, 161, 162, 164, 166, 198, 199
Jumping Jacks, etc. 55, 105, 135, 152

K

Katz, Rebecca (Integrative nutritionist) 192
Khurana, Sanjay 26, 61, 73, 75, 86–88, 91, 95, 97, 101, 106, 111, 112, 124, 126, 133, 140, 171, 188, 189, 200–204
Kyphosis (spine curvature) 40

L

Laminectomy 3, 99, 125, 126
Laparoscopic surgery 46
Lateral 218, 219
Legs (pain or lack of sensation) 13, 25, 36, 38, 69
Legumes (nutrition) 184, 185, 192, 193
Ligaments 76
Limitations (accepting and dealing with) 47, 114, 128, 134, 150, 196
Limp 6, 10, 53, 92, 107, 133, 141, 157, 202
Lind, James 177
Linda B. (patient) 20, 21, 45, 51, 52, 64, 65, 115–117, 129, 130, 159, 160, 186, 187
Lucio D. (patient) 24, 25, 46, 68–70, 72, 115, 117, 118, 132, 150, 168, 187, 195–197
Lumbar 6, 9, 10, 15, 25, 26, 76, 91

M

Mack Newton (educator, trainer) 12, 13, 90, 106
Magic-mineral-broth 192
Malnutrition 178
Manning, Peyton 72, 133
Manuka 136, 151, 152, 183
McDonalds (food) 182, 205
Mechanical (fixes) 30, 62, 79, 124, 201, 216
Medical device companies 1, 14, 74, 221, 222
Medical professionals 1, 2, 11, 32, 40, 44, 68, 103, 158, 209
Metabolism 185
Metamucil 137
Microbiome, microbiota, (gut health) 143, 183, 186, 190–193, 209
Micro-instability 98
Mind-body 158
Mindset (negative) 14, 67, 74, 95, 167, 186, 207

Mindset (positive) 11, 13, 14, 18, 78, 87, 93-95, 122, 123, 129, 139, 144, 148, 157, 158, 160, 168, 169, 171-173, 186, 198, 199, 201, 205, 207, 208

Minimally invasive 74, 83, 93, 125

Misinformation on the internet 68

Mobility challenges 2, 31, 112, 157, 202, 203, 214

Muscles, muscle-related 10, 25, 55, 56, 70, 76, 91, 104, 105, 135, 152-154, 217

MyPlate (Harvard) 181, 187, 206, 207, 209

N

Narcotics 93, 129, 137

Natural 8-10, 21, 59, 72, 130, 151, 180, 187

Nestle, Marion (nutritionist) 181

Neurogenic bladder 10, 53

Neurosurgery 99

Nightmare surgeries 73

Non-impact aerobic 102, 210

Non-invasive procedure 40

Non-opioid medication 167

Non-surgical options 60, 65

Normal function 3, 12, 27, 88, 137, 201

Nourishing your body 130, 209

Nutrition 6, 7, 9, 15, 46, 78, 102, 108, 116, 136, 138, 139, 144, 158, 159, 174, 176, 178-180, 182, 183, 186-190, 192, 205, 209, 210

Nutritional 7, 10, 115, 144, 179, 188, 190

Nutritionist 17, 47, 186, 187, 192, 211

Nuvasive (medical devices) 74, 125

O

Obese 191

Oldways (Mediterranean diet) 184

Operation 4, 9, 16, 43, 44, 79, 89, 99, 122, 139, 198, 214, 217, 221

Opioids 8, 9, 136, 143, 164, 165, 167, 179, 208, 209, 217, 220

Optimize 1-4, 6-13, 15, 17, 18, 33, 45-47, 53, 55, 65, 66, 73, 75, 77, 83, 85, 95, 96, 101-104, 107, 111-113, 115-122, 128, 138, 142, 143, 160, 168, 171, 172, 175, 178, 180, 188, 193, 201-204, 206-211, 213, 222, 225

Orthopedic 30, 31, 55, 64, 104

Osteoarthritis 203

Over-the-counter 23, 49, 202, 208

Oxygen 92, 120

P

Pain-free 1, 2, 12, 28, 78, 103, 128, 140, 169, 199

Painkiller 49, 70, 136, 143, 164-167, 208, 217, 220

Paleo 176

Pathology 74, 78, 79, 91, 95, 202

Pathways 136, 218

Patient-bill-rights 124

Pharmaceutical 7, 165

Physiological 111, 185

Phytochemicals (for healing) 184, 185

Postoperative 2, 9, 15, 16, 31, 110, 112, 138, 141, 158, 164, 175, 180, 187, 189, 218

Pregnancy 45, 48

Pre-habilitation 6, 31, 32, 55, 56, 60, 103, 104, 106, 107, 110–113, 134, 135, 157, 160, 172, 178, 210

Pre-operative 15, 16, 60, 101, 109, 110, 125, 204, 210

Preparation leads to improved outcomes 61, 106, 109, 112, 120, 168, 183, 207, 214

Prescription 10, 70, 179, 209, 220

Pritikin (Diet) 176

Probiotics 137, 143, 190, 192

Professional athletes 13, 32, 225

Programmed to heal 11, 16, 65, 103, 173

Psychological 14, 74, 75, 77, 218, 219

Pyramid (food) 180, 181, 184

Q

Quarry, Nate "Rock" 144–146, 158, 197, 198, 211, 223, 225

R

Radiographic 79

Recipe for a full recovery 157

Recipes for healing 175, 209

Recovering (from surgery) 2, 17, 31, 133, 141, 161, 163, 168, 178, 204, 207, 211

Regimen, exercise 60, 106, 109, 110, 115, 143, 188, 220

Rehabilitation 6, 10, 11, 31, 48, 55, 56, 78, 104, 105, 107, 110, 112–114, 134, 135, 137–142, 148, 150, 151, 153–158, 160, 163, 172, 178, 186, 208, 210

Relaxers (muscle) 25, 70, 217

Relieving pain 7, 55

Rest 4, 11, 25, 27, 33, 68, 102, 134, 137, 146, 159, 160, 165, 167, 200, 205, 206, 208–210, 217

Results 15, 32, 40, 54, 83, 86, 94, 107, 141, 147, 199

Retirement 81, 82, 162, 199

Robbins, Tony 158

Robert G. (patient, retiree) 21, 22, 28, 44, 56, 57, 65, 81, 115, 156, 162–164, 193, 199, 207

Rodman, Adam 33, 102, 210

S

Sauerkraut (probiotic) 191

Scoliosis 27, 42, 88, 98, 125

Scurvy 177, 178

Seeds (diet) 184, 192

Shoe horn (long) 222

Shoulder 42, 154

Shower (after care) 214–216, 220–222

Sinek, Simon 158

Singer, Blair 147

Skovrlj, Branko 29, 30, 76, 78, 86, 87, 92, 94, 95, 99, 100, 107–109, 112–114, 122, 128–129, 160, 169, 189–190, 204

Sleep 12, 33, 58, 81, 136, 165, 174, 209, 215, 222

Sogaard, Patti (MPT) 31, 66, 112–114, 128, 141, 150, 151, 166, 167, 172

Spasm (how to avoid) 155

Specialist 10, 42, 53, 59, 61, 64, 104, 131, 164, 203

Spices (dietary) 184

Spinal cord 25, 39, 91, 97, 124, 135

Spinal fusion 14, 20, 45, 149, 223

Spine surgeon(s) 4, 14, 17, 21, 28, 29, 39, 46, 49, 52, 53, 60-62, 64-67, 75, 80, 83, 97, 99, 101, 107, 160, 202

Spine surgery 1-3, 11, 13, 14, 16-18, 30-34, 40, 47-49, 51-53, 56, 57, 67, 68, 73, 76, 79, 80, 83, 85, 95-97, 99, 101-103, 106, 115, 121, 124, 141-144, 168, 169, 173, 175, 178-180, 183, 193, 199, 201, 210, 211, 213, 214, 222

Spondylolisthesis, Degenerative 27, 88

Standpoint of patient 8, 111, 127, 171, 172

Stanford University 74

Stenosis 27, 61, 67, 88, 89

Steroid shot 21, 52

Stiffness (pain) 32, 113

Stool softeners 9, 136

Stress 104, 117, 185, 205, 208, 221

Stretch 21, 22, 44, 52, 60, 71, 110, 119, 163-165, 187, 196

Sugar (effects of) 118, 136, 176, 190, 192, 193, 206

Suicide 29, 41

Suppository 143

Sweets 136, 184

Swim, swimming (aqua therapy) 11, 31, 35, 55, 67, 104, 134, 153, 159, 163, 210

Symptoms 26, 62, 73, 75, 79, 88, 101, 127

Syracuse University 174, 179, 180, 209

T

Techniques 2, 60, 83, 110, 124, 139, 142

Teton Orthopedics 30

TheOptimizedPatient.com 16

Therapeutic exercise 11, 136, 152, 153

Trauma (spinal) 16, 20, 21, 26, 31, 38, 40, 45-47, 73, 106, 111, 112, 136, 150, 178, 181, 200, 206, 207

Treatment 10, 30, 40, 54, 59, 61-64, 66, 78, 79, 89, 102, 112, 138, 140, 151, 177, 191, 196, 204, 210, 219

Trial and error 9, 141, 177, 224

Tumors 98, 125

Twain, Mark 14

Twist (refrain from) 3, 48, 146, 214-216, 220

U

Ultimate fighting championship 223

Unbearable pain 70

Undiagnosed degenerative disc disease 22

Urinary 27, 53

V

Vegetables 117, 118, 175, 177, 178, 180, 182, 184, 185, 187, 191-193, 205

Vegetarian 182, 192, 207

Vertebrae 20, 25, 39, 40

Vicious cycle 162

Visceral structures 126

Vitamin 108, 177, 178, 190

W

Walk, walking, walked 12, 26, 27, 34, 38, 44, 46, 49, 65, 69, 90, 97, 103, 106, 110, 114, 116, 117, 124, 134, 135, 140, 141, 148, 153, 155, 157, 159, 160, 162, 186, 187, 197, 202, 214, 216

Walton, Bill (NBA all-star) 8, 11, 32, 104, 124

Warren, Wileen 220

Wealth = health 211

Weekly coaching via video 115, 188

Weight 36, 85, 102, 104–106, 152, 171, 176, 179, 180, 182, 193, 205–207, 210

Well-informed decision 17

Western medicine 7

Wetsuit (for aqua therapy) 156

Wheelchair 27, 68, 90, 96, 153, 155, 166, 201, 202

Willett, Walter 181

Wish I had known before... 56, 106, 130

Women (deal with pain) 93

Workout buddy 18

X

XLIF 125, 144

X-ray 19, 22, 39, 42, 63, 69, 73, 106

Y

Yogurt 184, 191

YouTube 80, 119

Made in the USA
Monee, IL
04 November 2026

67387506R00144